MEDICAL REVOLUTIONARIES

KAROL K. WEAVER

Medical Revolutionaries

THE ENSLAVED HEALERS OF
EIGHTEENTH-CENTURY
SAINT DOMINGUE

UNIVERSITY OF ILLINOIS PRESS

URBANA AND CHICAGO

∞ This book is printed on acid-free paper.

Library of Congress Cataloging-in-Publication Data

Weaver, Karol K. (Karol Kimberlee)
Medical revolutionaries : the enslaved healers of
eighteenth-century Saint Domingue / Karol K. Weaver.
p. cm.
Includes bibliographical references and index.
ISBN-13: 978-0-252-03085-7 (cloth : alk. paper)
ISBN-10: 0-252-03085-0 (cloth : alk. paper)
ISBN-13: 978-0-252-07321-2 (pbk.: alk. paper)
ISBN-10: 0-252-07321-5 (pbk.: alk. paper)
1. Medicine—History—18th century. 2. Healing—Haiti—
History—18th century. 3. Slaves—Medicine—Haiti—
History—18th century. 4. Blacks—Medicine—Haiti—
History—18th century. I. Title.
[DNLM: 1. Delivery of Health Care—history—Haiti.
2. Medicine, Traditional—history—Haiti. 3. Social
Problems—history—Haiti. 4. Politics—Haiti. 5. African
Continental Ancestry Group—history—Haiti. 6. History,
18th Century—Haiti. WZ 70 DH2 W363m 2006]
R475.H2W43   2006
610.97294—dc22   2005035178

For Paul

Contents

Illustrations

Acknowledgments

A book is never the work of a single individual but results from the labor of strangers, teachers, friends, and family. I owe a word of thanks to the many librarians and archivists who assisted me. I received excellent service from the personnel at the Archives Nationales in Paris, the Archives d'Outre-mer in Aix-en-Provence, the Hagley Museum and Library in Wilmington, Delaware, the College of Physicians of Philadelphia, the Library Company of Philadelphia, the American Philosophical Society of Philadelphia, the Rare Books Room at Haverford College, the Rare Books Room at Pattee Library at the Pennsylvania State University, the Newberry Library, and the Blough-Weis Library at Susquehanna University. Many institutions and organizations generously provided funding: the Camargo Foundation, the Institut Français de Washington, the Hagley Museum and Library, the Francis Wood Institute at the College of Physicians of Philadelphia, the Research and Graduate Studies Office and the Department of History at the Pennsylvania State University, the School of Liberal Arts at Purdue University, and the Office of the Provost at Susquehanna University. Sections of the book include material from an article, "The Enslaved Healers of Eighteenth-Century Saint Domingue," that first appeared in the *Bulletin of the History of Medicine,* and from an article, " 'She Crushed the Child's Fragile Skull': Disease, Infanticide, and Enslaved Women in Eighteenth-Century Saint-Domingue," which appeared in its entirety in the journal *French Colonial History* 5 (2004), published by Michigan State University Press.

William V. Hudon helped me when I was an undergraduate, a graduate student, and a colleague with his generosity, advice, and friendship.

John B. Frantz taught me what it is to be an excellent teacher. Nancy Gabin was both a friend and a mentor. Bernard Moitt answered my questions, and Laurent Dubois helped me improve my work. Londa Schiebinger was a fine graduate adviser. Joan Catapano was an excellent editor.

Finally, family encouraged me, motivated me, and sustained me. My sister Kaleen Kovalovich gave so willingly of her goodness that I will never repay my debts to her. My sister Krisa Moncavage cheered me and advised me. My brother Kurt Kovalovich willingly and happily listened to my stories. Lil and Andy Kovalovich raised and taught their children well. My mom's encouraging "just get it done" was a great motivator. I send all my love to my beautiful son Jonah. My husband and my best friend Paul Weaver supported, encouraged, and loved me. I dedicate this book to him.

MEDICAL REVOLUTIONARIES

Introduction

The traditional history of Western bio-medicine hails the work of medical revolutionaries like Ignaz Semmelweis, Louis Pasteur, and Joseph Lister. These men stepped outside the narrow confines of the medicine of their day and instituted changes that transformed how the world thought and practiced medicine. No less important are the enslaved healers of eighteenth-century Saint Domingue. Enslaved healers such as *hospitalières, infirmières, accoucheuses* (midwives), herbalists, veterinary practitioners, and *kaperlatas* existed and flourished in the medical world of Saint Domingue. Although history recorded few of their names, the influence that they had on medicine and society in Saint Domingue and elsewhere was tremendous. Their work had significant social, medical, economic, and political consequences for slaves as well as for their European and Creole masters.

Using Western, African, and Caribbean remedies, enslaved healers treated their fellow slaves, white residents, and nonhuman animals. They enabled thousands of slaves to survive another day, or at least to die comforted with the familiarity of traditional African medical techniques. In the midst of a life-threatening and soul-crushing labor system, these men and women searched through the wilds of Saint Domingue, identified new plants, experimented with them, and created new medical systems that joined Western medicine, African herbalism, and Caribbean medical care.

Moreover, the enslaved healers were excellent practitioners of medicine—they were able to retain a large clientele and profit from their healing strategies. They realized that herbal remedies appealed to not only their fellow slaves, but also to the white men and women they served. They understood the power and profitability of healing rituals. They comprehended that the populace they served, including both whites and blacks, depended on both the physical and the spiritual solace that medicine provided.

What is more significant, the enslaved healers of eighteenth-century Saint Domingue created an ideology and system of resistance that included sabotage, the taking of both human and nonhuman life, and terrorism. This ideology and system of resistance inspired some of the most important figures of the Haitian Revolution. In order to fully understand the origins and impact of the Haitian Revolution, one must comprehend that the enslaved healers emerged as significant leaders of slave communities through a process of cultural retention, assimilation, and creation, profited economically and politically from their healing practices, and initiated and implemented an ideology of resistance via sabotage and the destruction of human and animal life.

The labor undertaken by enslaved healers allowed them to retain elements of African healing traditions, to appropriate Western and Caribbean medical techniques, and to contribute to the creation of an Afro-Caribbean health care system. Their work as enslaved healers echoed African social roles. They combined traditional knowledge with Caribbean and Western healing techniques in order to formulate medical systems more closely attuned to the health needs of a population that struggled under the physical and psychological burdens of slavery. Like African females before them, *hospitalières* (women who were in charge of plantation hospitals) and *infirmières* (hospital aids) played a part in inoculation procedures that attempted to preserve their fellow slaves from debility, disfigurement, and even death brought on by smallpox. They also utilized African remedies in their treatment of slaves who suffered from *pian* (yaws) and *maladies vermineuses* (parasites). By assimilating Western humoral therapy into their healing repertoire, the *hospitalières* created new medical systems and were able to offer their patients diverse types of medical care. Whether they wanted to or not, *hospitalières, infirmières,* and midwives learned to work under the authority of male plantation surgeons and in Western-inspired lying-in institutions.

Like the *hospitalières, infirmières,* and midwives, herbalists offered to African and Creole slaves plant remedies that were more familiar than the medicines distributed by the master and his white employees. Herbalists drew upon African herbalism as they ministered to patients enduring wounds, fevers, and scurvy. They utilized traditional remedies like baths, salves, and lotions but prepared them from plants they found in Saint Domingue. Not content and often not able to simply employ African medical therapeutics, enslaved herbalists incorporated remedies from the Caribbean pharmacopoeia and, in the process, created an Afro-Caribbean medical system.

Similarly, mesmerists, veterinary artists, and *kaperlatas* (practitioners of spiritual and natural medicine) looked to African divination for inspiration. The European magnetist craze as well as Caribbean medico-religious rituals influenced the work of the enslaved mesmerists. Through the appropriation of these forms of spiritual healing, slaves created a Creole network of supernatural healers who sorted themselves according to their affiliation with *kaperlatas* and *macandalistes* (purveyors of charms and talismans).

In addition to using diverse therapies, enslaved healers emerged as leaders within slave communities; through the practice of medicine they gained both political and material power. *Hospitalières* and midwives occupied the most respected positions within the slave hierarchy; both whites and blacks identified them as the most significant female members of the enslaved community. In fact, *hospitalières* and midwives were the female equivalents of the *commandeurs,* the enslaved men responsible for supervising and driving their fellow slave laborers. *Hospitalières* and midwives benefited materially from the work they performed—they received extra food and clothing in exchange for the important service they provided. In addition, these women, like many other enslaved domestics, had a greater opportunity to be granted or to gain their freedom, probably the most important way for an African or Afro-Caribbean slave to improve his or her economic and social position in the racially divided colony of Saint Domingue.

Unlike *hospitalières* and midwives, herbalists, mesmerists, and *kaperlatas* existed outside the plantation labor hierarchy recognized by whites; nonetheless, they were leaders among enslaved men and women, who sought them out for the physical and cultural comfort they dispensed. This leadership translated into financial gain. Herbalists, most especially female market women, profited from the sale of herbal concoctions in the colonial marketplaces. Mesmerists and *kaperlatas* benefited from the charms and talismans they sold. The money that the enslaved healers accumulated presented them with the opportunity to purchase many items, including extra food and clothing and, most important, weapons and freedom.

Enslaved healers also participated in occupational sabotage; in other words, they used their positions to interfere with the productivity of the plantation and the work completed there. Ultimately, occupational sabotage resulted in physical violence and the destruction of human and animal life. Terror was one of the basic characteristics of occupational sabotage. Enslaved healers who assumed power were willing to foster allegiance through intimidation. Slaves who did not remain loyal took the chance of being killed.

Hospitalières played a part in occupational sabotage by allowing malingerers to remain within the walls of the plantation hospital long after their real or feigned illnesses had been cured. After caring for the sick for many years, *hospitalières* easily differentiated between the truly ill and those feigning illness. Their complicity in acts of deception compounded the negative consequences for the master. The slave was not working, needed rest was made available to the malingerer, and extra food and medicines were expended. The high rank that the *hospitalière* held meant that she could demand food and supplies from the planter's storehouse. Moreover, the psychological satisfaction that both "patient" and *hospitalière* received from deceiving the master or his employee was, no doubt, exhilarating. *Hospitalières* had access to European medicines that could easily be turned on the master and his family, but more often on his livestock and on his slaves.

Midwives and *infirmières* also had ample opportunity to engage in occupational sabotage. Enslaved midwives explored the wilderness that surrounded their plantations for plants, like the avocado tree, that might be used to procure abortions for desperate slave mothers. Their discovery and application of various plants also provided women with the means to end the suffering of newborn infants through the practice of infanticide. Through their work as *commandeuses*, *infirmières* had control over the labor of the third field gang and could limit the productivity of this group as needed.

Herbalists provided concoctions leading to death. By serving as diviners, *kaperlata*s and magnetizers promised their clients protection from harm perpetrated by disloyal blacks and cruel whites. Due to the high level of independence and trust accorded them by their masters, veterinary practitioners had greater freedom of movement. They had the opportunity to meet secretly with fellow revolutionaries. They also possessed knowledge of plants, which they used to poison both human and nonhuman animals. Eventually, these enslaved healers became legendary figures whose inspiration, ideas, and activities fueled the revolution that led to freedom for the enslaved men and women of Saint Domingue.

The story of the healers of Saint Domingue will add to the history of enslaved medical practitioners in the New World, a subject that has been taking shape over the last several decades. Richard Sheridan introduced his readers to the various healers who worked in the British West Indies. He noted the important work done by midwives and hothouse workers, or the men and women who cared for ailing slaves in plantation hospitals. Sheridan also studied *obeah* practitioners, male and female slaves who sold drugs, poisons, and charms.[1] In her book on health, disease, and medical care in nineteenth-century Martinique, Geneviève Leti discussed the duties of *hospitalières*, midwives, and *infirmières* and analyzed the variety of services provided by local empirics.[2] Todd Savitt and Katherine Bankole completed historical studies of enslaved healers in the American South.[3]

Accounts of healing by enslaved men and women in eighteenth-century Saint Domingue also have been compiled. The best-known study is that of French historian Pierre Pluchon, who argued that the French focused their legislative efforts on a class of healers known as sorcerers. He analyzed how French notions of sorcery influenced the perceptions of Africans as practitioners of black magic and malicious medicine. He also established a connection between French perceptions of vodou and the legal prohibitions against the practice of medicine among slaves and people of color. Finally, Pluchon considered the documented instances of poisoning in Saint Domingue, the reaction of vigilante whites to these events, and the attempts by Europeans (specifically, physicians and Jesuits) to defend Africans and Afro-Caribbeans from charges of sorcery and poisoning.[4]

Other writers touch briefly on the existence of fringe medical practitioners. Gabriel Debien focused his efforts on the responsibilities of female slave health care providers, especially the duties of the *hospitalière*. He also referred to remedies employed by slave herbalists but did not pursue the topic except to say that these medical therapies are recorded in eighteenth-century travel books.[5] In his classic study of science and medicine in Saint Domingue, James McClellan mentioned that healers catered to the health needs of the nonwhite population, noted their outlaw status, and briefly discussed the *kaperlata* and the condemnations brought against this type of healer by members of the medical establishment.[6] More recently, McClellan and François Regourd have collaborated on an article that describes the scientific and medical administration of the colony and the existence of marginal health practitioners like the enslaved healers.[7] Bernard Moitt studied slave women who worked as *hospitalières* and midwives and observed that the "role of black females in the health care arena has been minimized in the literature on slavery, and their functions have usually been ill defined, if at all."[8] Despite the impressive work completed by these authors, they did not focus on the variety of practitioners nor did they note the contributions that slaves made to the revolution that ultimately freed Saint Domingue from French control and resulted in the establishment of the Haitian Republic.

This work also fits into recent debates over our understanding of the history of tropical medicine. David Arnold's introduction to *Warm Climates and Western Medicine* noted that the traditional history of tropical medicine emphasizes the work of Patrick Manson and the development of the medical specialty in the late nineteenth century. Arnold and his fellow researchers argue that long before the late nineteenth century other physicians, scientists, and common men and women completed important work through their study of the diseases and medicine of the "warm climates" or "the Torrid Zone." These common men and women included the enslaved healers of eighteenth-century Saint Domingue.[9]

This book is motivated by two major theoretical concerns. First, the story of the enslaved healers responds to an important question I encountered when studying the history of slavery: how did the activities of slaves simultaneously support and resist the slave system?[10] Some writers see acts of cultural retention, assimilation, and creation as types of resistance strategies, while others perceive them as encouraging accommodation.[11] Specifically, Hilary Beckles, Bernard Moitt, and Jennifer Morgan recognize the formation of cultural systems as integral elements of survival and resistance.[12] My reading of the enslaved healers tends toward the interpretations of accommodation and resistance put forward by Beckles, Moitt, and Morgan. The enslaved healers' pattern of resistance incorporated a great many techniques with which to oppose slavery and white rule. They developed an Afro-Caribbean medical system, took part in Afro-Caribbean religious ceremonies, ran away, practiced infanticide and abortion, poisoned people and animals, carried and used agricultural implements as weapons, kept healthy slaves and animals from working by confining them in hospitals, and expended food and medical supplies. Narratives of resistance in Saint Domingue tend to emphasize marronage and vodou as key elements of insurgence and downplay other forms of rebellion and resistance.[13] The enslaved healers did use *marronage* and participated in vodou, but, as David Geggus has argued, slave rebels such as the enslaved healers also used other means to organize and bring their dream of freedom to fruition.[14] My understanding of acts of resistance is informed by the work of James Scott, who recognized that "the aggregation of thousands upon thousands of such 'petty' acts of resistance have dramatic economic and political effects."[15] In the case of Saint Domingue, resistance undertaken by enslaved healers helped to topple a slave system and led to the loss of France's most significant and productive New World colony. In addition, the defeats that Napoleon sustained as a result of the Haitian Revolution led to political decisions that affected France's presence on the North American continent and the history of the United States.

The story of resistance by enslaved healers also places enslaved women in more central roles than prior histories, which have focused on the roles of slave drivers in revolt, and in so doing expands our understanding of women's roles in plantation life and slave resistance. Studying the actions undertaken by the enslaved healers contributes to the burgeoning literature on the subject of women's participation in slavery and slave resistance that has been completed by scholars such as Beckles, Moitt, Morgan, and Barbara Bush.[16] In particular, *hospitalières, infirmières,* midwives, *pacotilleurs* (peddlers), and the *kaperlatas* forcefully and skillfully resisted slavery.

A second theoretical concern of this book is the use of a new type of methodology called historical ethnomedicine, or the search for traditional medical techniques and remedies via primary sources, the verbal and nonverbal evidence used by historians. This new approach joins history with diverse disciplines such as the human medical sciences, the veterinary sciences, pharmacology, and anthropology. Due to the paucity of material left by the enslaved healers themselves, the historian investigating their practices must watch for them and listen for their voices in the texts and documents of eighteenth-century writers. The researcher as well as the reader needs to be aware of the ways French doctors, travel book authors, and colonists thought about medicine, healing, the body, disease, and race in order to understand the story of the enslaved healers. Thus, the book will not only emphasize the enslaved healers, but also the perspectives and prejudices of eighteenth-century authors who wrote about them. This strategy will demonstrate the complex dialogue and struggle between various colonial medical practitioners and the fissures and debates within the medical discourse of the period. In so doing, the author hopes to reveal the complicated and truly Atlantic medical worlds of the eighteenth century.

By necessity, the sources on which this study is based are rich and varied. Eighteenth-century medical books that analyze the disease environment of Saint Domingue are the foundation of my work. One example is Jean-Barthélemy Dazille's *Observations sur les maladies des nègres, leurs causes, leurs traitemens et les moyens de les prévenir,* a source that explains what types of medical problems slaves experienced. These books also give glimpses into the medical underworld of Saint Domingue. Now and then, readers encounter an enslaved healer and the remedies that he or she utilized.

Travel accounts also provided information about the customs, climate, and social life of Saint Domingue. Probably the most significant contribution to my study of enslaved healers is Nicolas Louis Bourgeois's

Voyages Intéressans dans Différentes Colonies, which details the herbal remedies used by enslaved healers to combat disease and heal wounds. The most important account of life in Saint Domingue is Médéric-Louis-Élie Moreau de Saint-Méry's multivolume masterpiece, *Description Topographique.*

Unpublished accounts include correspondence between plantation managers and absentee planters in France, plantation hospital records, and lists of slaves. These archival records document the health of female and male slaves and provide a grounds-eye view of medical treatment in Saint Domingue. In their correspondence, plantation managers tell their employers about the work completed by herbalists, *hospitalières, infirmières,* midwives, and veterinary practitioners.

Periodicals like the *Affiches Américaines* indicate the health issues that concerned literate residents, supply information about medical facilities staffed by slaves, and furnish popular accounts of healers. Another important publication was Duchemin de L'Étang's *Gazette de Médecine pour les Colonies,* the first medical journal in Saint Domingue, which described inoculation procedures undertaken by enslaved healers.

Court proceedings and compilations of medical legislation detail legal actions taken against enslaved healers. Moreau de Saint-Méry again provides an essential source of information with his comprehensive *Lois et Constitutions.* Likewise, Charles Arthaud's *Observations sur les Lois concernant la Médecine et la Chirurgie dans le Colonie de Saint-Domingue* gives a history of medical legislation, recounts the duties and responsibilities of official medical practitioners, and mentions the work of several types of enslaved healers.

Finally, the landscape of modern Haiti, with its dusty, unpaved roads, beautiful, breathtaking mountains, and wide stretches of beach, taught me about the allure of Saint Domingue, but also about its hidden recesses where many forms of medicine could be and are still practiced today. Country doctors, men and women who provide medical care to their neighbors, continue to employ herbal remedies that were used by enslaved herbalists in the eighteenth century. Medicines are still cultivated in gardens, collected, and utilized to treat conditions similar to those that devastated the slave population. Like the enslaved healers, country doctors profit economically and politically from their healing. Like the slaves, the patients of these traditional healers react to the convergence of unlike medical systems with conflicted emotions. They realize the dangers that a competing medical system presents to a community and its culture and respond to these challenges with a mixture of gratitude, resignation, and hostility.

Along with the secondary sources compiled by historians and other scholars, these primary sources have proven invaluable in helping to craft the intriguing story of the enslaved healers. In the following pages, I will be relating the history of Saint Domingue, its official medical establishment, and the medical world created by the enslaved healers. Chapter 1 highlights the colony of Saint Domingue under French rule. Known as the "Pearl of the Antilles," Saint Domingue was the most important and most productive French colony of the eighteenth century. The paradisiacal image of the island was balanced by its reputation as the Torrid Zone, a place of danger, disease, and death. This chapter provides an overview of the geography, society, and economy of Saint Domingue and a description of the colony's racial system and its dependence on slavery. Finally, the chapter will analyze the disease demographics of the island and the reasons for the high incidence of disease.

Chapter 2 investigates the official practice of medicine that existed in order to define disease and to fight it. The official practitioners of medicine held great economic, social, and political power in Saint Domingue. They were responsible for suggesting public health legislation; fighting disease on slaving ships, in prisons, and on plantations; and regulating and licensing their fellow medical men and women. Unable to deal with the diseases they encountered in Saint Domingue and driven by economic and professional ambition, many practitioners turned to the enslaved healers for medical remedies.

Chapter 3 introduces readers to life on a Saint Domingue plantation and the enslaved women who served as medical care providers for their fellow slaves and their white masters. These women—the *hospitalière*, the *infirmière*, and the *accoucheuse*—were respected and valuable members of the slave hierarchy whose medical skills were exploited for the economic gain of plantation managers and to combat abolitionist agitation in France. Yet the *hospitalières*, *infirmières*, and midwives actively undermined and resisted slavery by retaining African medical traditions, fashioning an Afro-Caribbean health system, assuming leadership roles in their community, allowing those pretending to be ill to remain within the plantation hospital to avoid work, providing infant care to expectant mothers, supplying the same women with abortions, and participating in acts of infanticide.

The role of the herbalists in the creation of an Afro-Caribbean or Creole pharmacopoeia is the focus of chapter 4. The search by French and Creole medical practitioners for information from these African and Afro-Caribbean men and women provides evidence that non-Western medical knowledge was appropriated and incorporated into the Western medical corpus. Yet the whites of Saint Domingue nervously eyed the herbalists because along with their ability to heal came the potential to harm as well.

Chapter 5 presents the history of the enslaved veterinary practitioners. Their work was essential to the economy of Saint Domingue, which depended on animals as a source of food and fuel. The main enslaved veterinary practitioners were the *gardiens de bêtes* and the *pacotilleurs.* Makandal, one of the most famous *gardiens de bêtes,* and his association with the *pacotilleurs* helped to inspire fellow slaves to resist their slave masters, overthrow French rule, and establish the Republic of Haiti.

Chapter 6 relates the story of the Saint Domingue mesmerists. The arrest of these magnetizers was an attack on healing undertaken by slaves and people of color as well as an assault on slaves who dared to oppose the white population. The slaves not only practiced what Saint Domingue authorities considered a bizarre form of therapy but also held secret nighttime meetings at which hundreds of slaves congregated. White residents saw mesmerist activity as the dangerous breakdown of hierarchy, the deterioration of social position, and the destruction of Saint Domingue's slave society. The enslaved supporters of magnetism saw it differently; for them, mesmerism offered freedom from established medicine, and what is more significant, freedom from the authority of the white master.

In the eyes of French and Creole officials, the *kaperlata*s, the main actors in chapter 7, were the most dangerous element of the medical underworld of eighteenth-century Saint Domingue. Initially considered akin to sorcerers, they practiced divination and distributed herbal remedies among slaves, people of color, and lower-class whites. In the midst of revolution, colonial authorities deemed them dangerous influences with the potential to destroy white society and grasp control of the island. Ultimately, the practices, power, and prestige associated with the *kaperlata* became so great that the term was subsumed by practitioners of vodou to identify a magical charm and the one who sold them.

1 Saint Domingue: Life in the Torrid Zone

> The French part of the island of Saint Domingue is, of all the possessions of France in the New World, the most important because of the wealth that it procures for its metropole and by the influence that it has on agriculture and commerce.
>
> —Médéric-Louis-Élie Moreau de Saint-Méry, *Description Topographique*, 1797

Between the breathtaking blue of the Caribbean Sea and the waters of the Atlantic Ocean lies Hispaniola, the island with which Christopher Columbus made contact in 1492. Mountains and plains dominate the island's landscape. The original Arawakan and Cariban inhabitants of the island possessed a political system governed by caciques. These leaders ruled over people gathered in villages along the coasts as well as inland. Ten or more families dwelled in wooden and thatch houses, which faced a larger building in which the local cacique lived and an open field where festivities and ceremonies took place. Residents cultivated both plant and animal life. They grew manioc and harvested turtles, large fish, and manatees from the sea and from large aquaculture ponds.

The encounter between these native Caribbeans and Europeans in 1492 had disastrous and devastating consequences for Hispaniola's residents. Once totaling more than three million people, the population of the island practically disappeared by 1570. The importation of disease—most especially the transmission of infectious ailments like measles and smallpox from Europeans to Native Caribbeans—facilitated Spanish conquest. Forced labor in Spanish-run mines also depleted the native population.[1]

French presence in the area emerged rather late. In 1629, *boucaniers*, Frenchmen whose name indicated their practice of roasting, grilling, and smoking meats, and *flibustiers*, individuals so-called because of their use of light sailing vessels, headquartered themselves on Tortuga, an island off the north coast of Saint Domingue.[2] By 1659, the adventurers came within France's sphere of influence. From Tortuga, they established settlements on Saint Domingue. With the signing of the Treaty of Ryswick in 1697, which ended the War of the Grand Alliance, the western half of the island came under the control of France while the eastern half remained the domain of Spain.[3]

Known as the Pearl of the Antilles, Saint Domingue was the most important French colony in the eighteenth century. Plantations produced three major cash crops: sugar, coffee, and indigo. In addition, the soils of Saint Domingue provided food for the local markets and feed for the livestock raised by colonial planters.[4] Most plantation owners lived in France and left the daily supervision of their landholdings to a variety of plantation employees, the most important being the *gérant* or plantation manager. Enslaved African, Afro-Caribbean, and biracial men and women performed the most strenuous labor on the plantations. The average plantation housed 200 slaves, but there are instances of landholdings where more than 1,000 slaves lived.[5]

Commercially, Saint Domingue was the linchpin of the French Empire; one French person in eight made a living by means of colonial trade. French cities like Nantes, Bordeaux, and Marseilles depended on their trade with the colony. Shipbuilding, slave trading, and sugar refining flourished in these urban centers as a result of contact with Saint Domingue. In addition, these areas supplied the colony with French-made as well as European-produced items such as cloth, salted meat, flour, dairy products, fruits, vegetables, wines, liquors, and hardware. Nantes, Bordeaux, and Marseilles also profited from the importation and sale of colonial products like coffee, sugar, cocoa, and hides.[6] The colony's main commercial ports were Port-au-Prince and, more important, Cap-François (also spelled Cap-Français; modern Cap-Haïtien), known as the Paris of the Antilles.[7]

Abiding by mercantilist policy, France saw its colonies as revenue producers. France hoped to profit from the sale of colonial goods both at home and abroad and through taxation. In order to achieve these goals, France subjected Saint Domingue to a monopoly—colonists bought items from France, sold their goods to France, and traded via French shippers. Smuggling negated France's total domination over Saint Domingue commerce.

Nevertheless, colonial economic policy affected social relations in the colonies; animosity existed between planters and colonial merchants. Planters generally complained about the high prices of imports, especially slaves, while the traders grumbled over the colonists' inability or refusal to repay debts.[8]

Being French subjects, the colonists came under the legal authority of the customs of Paris and the edicts enacted by the monarchy in France. The Minister of the Marine, also known as the Minister of the Colonies, directed and superintended all colonial affairs at the request of the French monarch and was advised by two boards of agriculture, one in Cap-François and one in Port-au-Prince, the members of which made recommendations to the minister and also submitted reports after the departures or deaths of the governor and *intendant*.[9] The governor was a military officer who normally ruled for a term of three years, controlled the army, and acted as the official representative of the French monarch. The *intendant* oversaw legal, financial, and administrative matters. Commissioners assisted the *intendant* by providing information about finances, troop inspections, hospital assessments, and control of the warehouses.[10] Together, the governor and the *intendant* enacted laws, appointed officials, and distributed land. They also headed two *conseils supérieurs* located in Port-au-Prince and Cap-François; by 1787, these two courts were joined to form a single court, the *Conseil Supérieur de Saint Domingue*.[11] Although the common law of Paris and laws enacted by the king were the legal foundations of the colony, these colonial courts created laws, registered royal edicts, and served as appeals courts for decisions made by provincial tribunals.[12] The governor, *intendant*, military officers, and provincial officials regulated the colony's income. The division of the colony into three provinces, the west, south, and north, aided political administration. Each province came under the authority of a lieutenant governor and a tribunal of justice and possessed a *sénéchaussée* (or militia), which was responsible for maintaining law and order.[13] Because political leaders and their armed forces resided in the urban areas, law enforcement was difficult. Abbé Guillaume Raynal noted, "There are two governments in Saint Domingue whose principles are very different; one is the public authority while the other is domestic authority."[14] The isolation that characterized plantation life checked the power of political administrators to execute laws and punish offenders.

The Roman Catholic Church also played a part in the political administration of the colony. An apostolic prefect, appointed by the king, chose parish priests who generally possessed a piece of land and several slaves owned by the church. The priests contributed to the maintenance of law and order by offering an ideology and way of life to which colonists and their slaves might submit. Unfortunately for them, their power to in-fluence law and order was affected negatively by corruption, disease, and indifference. Former coffee planter and member of the *Conseil Supérieur* P. J. Laborie said there was "a general contempt of religion, and profligacy of manners, . . . fatal and unfortunate circumstances in our colonies."[15] Tempted by the substantial property that the church owned and by the money paid them by the king, priests lost the respect of the people as a result of their ignorance and avarice. In order to combat these moral fail-ings, the vicar, governor, and *intendant* had the power to send corrupt members of the clergy back to France. Spiritual bankruptcy was made worse by the inability of priests to fight off disease. Two of the major re-ligious orders who served the colony, the Dominicans and the Capuchins, were unable to furnish replacements for those priests who succumbed to illness.[16] Northern Saint Domingue, for example, had been under the re-ligious influence of the Capuchins, but after they were unable to field enough religious, the Jesuits, who were well known for their efforts to reach out to slaves and discourage them from their so-called superstitious practices, then assumed control of the area's religious destiny. By the 1760s, the Jesuit order was expelled. This event was not unique to Saint Domingue; worldwide efforts to eradicate the Society of Jesus had begun in 1759 and came to a head in 1773 when Pope Clement XIV suppressed the order.[17] Nevertheless, the colonists welcomed the removal of the Je-suits from the island because of their proselytizing efforts among the slaves. One Jesuit in Cap-François became notorious for teaching slaves; his work was vilified, not praised.[18] After the removal of the Jesuits, the Dominicans and Capuchins remained to shepherd the faithful. The in-difference of planters to their own religious edification and that of their slaves limited the power of the priests. Despite their shortcomings, mem-bers of the religious life provided important services to the colonists. A convent of nuns in Cap-François educated young girls, while the Broth-ers of Charity tended the sick at the Royal Hospital in Cap-François.[19]

Socially, Saint Domingue was divided by race into three major cate-gories, *blancs* (whites), *affranchis* (free men and women of color or bira-cial descent), and *esclaves* (slaves). Whites, who made up only 6% of the total population in Saint Domingue, were separated further by class stand-ing and their place of origin.[20] The *grands blancs* (great whites), including large-scale plantation owners, French maritime officials, and French-born bureaucrats, enjoyed a greater degree of economic, social, and political power than the *petits blancs* (little whites), such as small farmers, soldiers, sailors, shopkeepers, white servants, and whites who lived among and with nonwhites. Over time, persons of more middling status, such as successful medical practitioners and high-ranking plantation employees, also came to be included among the "great whites" of Saint Domingue. Well aware of the class bias among members of the white population, slaves developed their own system of titles for members of these groups that played into the racism upon which colonial society was built. They called whites of the upper class *blancs-blancs* (white whites), while whites of the lower class were identified disparagingly as *blanchets* (little whites) and *faux blancs* (fake whites). Slaves reserved their highest contempt for white militiamen or the *nègres-blancs* (black whites).[21]

Whites also were separated by their place of origin. The term *Créole* (Creole) referred to men and women who were born in Saint Domingue or in another colony. The Creoles were distinguished from newly arrived Europeans or *transplantés*, who made up the largest percentage of the total white population in Saint Domingue. More than 75% of whites were immigrants from France with Gascony providing the largest share of settlers over the course of the eighteenth century.[22] The white immigrant population was overwhelmingly male, men outnumbering women twenty to one. Most male immigrants were unfettered by marriage. Besides being mostly male and single, the immigrant population of Saint Domingue was a transient group. Most new arrivals did not take the time to put down roots; instead, they hoped to make a quick fortune, pack up their gains, and head back to a comfortable life in France. Because they were few, European women are rarely mentioned in eighteenth-century books about the island.

The second racial category, the *affranchis* (free men and women of color) were a population known under a variety of names. The most famous chronicler of life in eighteenth-century Saint Domingue, Moreau de Saint-Méry, provided a summary of the designations when he wrote "The *Affranchis* are more universally known under the name of *Gens de couleur* or *Sang-mêlés*, although the term *Gens de couleur*, taken literally, also refers to the black slaves." The categorization of people into this class depended on whether a person had "black blood." Moreau de Saint-Méry separated people of mixed race into eleven groups based on the amount of white and black parentage they possessed (Figure 1). Moreau de Saint-Méry put the population of men and women of color at 28,000. As a result of being born in the colony, men and women of color fell under the category of Creole. This term, however, was not often used to describe them because their status as Creoles was understood.[23]

Due to the racism that prevailed in the colony, the law severely limited the rights of *affranchis*; they were unable to serve in the army or navy, practice law or medicine, become members of the clergy, and hold public

FRANÇAISE DE SAINT-DOMINGUE.   71

RÉSULTAT

De toutes les nuances, produites par les diverfes combinaifons du mélange des Blancs avec les Nègres, & des Nègres avec les Caraïbes ou Sauvages ou Indiens Occidentaux, & avec les Indiens Orientaux.

I.

Combinaifons du Blanc.

D'un Blanc & d'une	Négreffe, vient	un Mulâtre.
	Mulâtreffe,	Quarteron.
	Quarterone,	Métif.
	Métive,	Mamelouque.
	Mamelouque,	Quarteronné.
	Quarteronnée,	Sang-mêlé.
	Sang-mêlée,	Sang-mêlé, qui s'approche continuellement du Blanc.
	Marabou,	Quarteron.
	Griffonne,	Quarteron.
	Sacatra,	Quarteron.

I I.

Combinaifons du Nègre.

D'un nègre & d'une	Blanche, vient	un Mulâtre.
	Sang-mêlée,	Mulâtre.
	Quarteronnée,	Mulâtre.
	Mamelouque,	Mulâtre.
	Métive,	Mulâtre.
	Quarteronne,	Marabou.
	Mulâtreffe,	Griffe.
	Marabou,	Griffe.
	Griffonne,	Sacatra.
	Sacatra,	Sacatra.

Figure 1. A section of Moreau de Saint-Méry's racial chart indicating the different "combinations" of interracial men and women. Moreau de Saint-Méry, Description Topographique *(Philadelphia, 1797), 1: 71. Used by permission of the American Philosophical Society.*

office. Over the course of the second half of the eighteenth century, colonial authorities prohibited them from wearing European clothes, carrying weapons, assembling, remaining in France, being addressed as *monsieur* and *madame,* and dining with white men and women. In spite of these restrictions and the disdain that whites had for men and women of

color, they prospered. They were well-known craftworkers and large property and slaveholders. The emphasis placed upon race in the colony of
Saint Domingue meant that the people of biracial and multiracial descent
looked upon the lowest social class, the slaves, with the highest contempt.[24]

The largest portion of the Saint Domingue population was made up
of *esclaves* (enslaved men and women). Approximately 452,000 slaves
lived and work in the French colony.[25] Slaves were separated into two
groups: the *nouveaux,* or slaves from western Africa, and Creole slaves,
or men and women who were born into slavery in the colony.

Race not only divided the residents of Saint Domingue; where one
lived also shaped one's destiny. Merchants, craftspeople, legal and political officials, physicians, sailors, and soldiers inhabited the urban areas.
City life in Saint Domingue offered them a number of diversions. The
colony was home to four theaters, the seating of which reinforced racial
division within the colony. Whites sat on the main floor and in boxes reserved for them; men and women of color, on the other hand, were limited to boxes. Those colonists interested in fashion consulted skilled
seamstresses of color, well known for their exquisite but expensive work.
Visitors to the colony could expect to find hotel service in the cities and
market towns.[26] For those colonists interested in cultivating the life of
the mind, Saint Domingue offered several libraries, a daily newspaper, and
a small but active medical and scientific community that was responsible for a steady stream of publications and the establishment of a colonial scientific academy known as the *Cercle des Philadelphes.* In addition, two royal printing houses existed, one in Cap-François and the other
in Port-au-Prince.[27]

Plantations dominated the countryside of Saint Domingue; planters,
their employees, and their slaves constituted its residents. Whites enjoyed
promenades along the seashore or on the roads that bordered the great
plantations. Men and women often stopped to admire the plantation gardens, which grew a beautiful and aromatic array of flowers and fruits. Due
to the lack of hotels in rural areas, travelers relied on the legendary hos-
pitality of planters and their employees. Market towns infiltrated the areas
between the city and countryside and were important gathering points
for slaves, who sold their extra produce there.[28]

The Torrid Zone

Saint Domingue's reputation as a profitable, productive, and pleasing location was balanced by the perception that the island was the epitome

of the Torrid Zone, a place of disease and death. The Torrid Zone, a geographic term, refers to one of the five zones into which the earth is divided. Geographers place the Torrid Zone between the Tropic of Cancer
and the Tropic of Capricorn. The other four regions are the northern and
southern Temperate Zones and the northern and southern Frigid Zones.
The partition of the globe into zones was the work of Greek philosophers,
in particular Aristotle, who employed the concept of the climatic zones
in order to comment on the habitability of the earth. According to Aristotle, the extreme heat of the Torrid Zone and the excessive cold of the
Frigid Zones made these areas uninhabitable.[29] Seventeenth-century author Jean-Baptiste Dutertre provided an excellent summary of the idea
when he wrote

> It is not without reason that the ancient Geographers . . . had believed not
> only that the regions situated under the extreme zones, that is it to say,
> under the Artic and Antarctic poles were uninhabitable, but even those
> that are under the middle zone, commonly called Torrid, . . . believing
> that the ice and continual cold caused by the distance of the sun, ren-
> dered these first two places uninhabitable; and that the second receive
> the same misfortune by the continual presence of this star, which by the
> devouring heat of its rays, burns and dries . . . to such an extent . . . , that
> it is incapable of maintaining habitants, animals, trees, or plants.[30]

Aristotle's notion continued to have supporters as well as detractors
in the seventeenth and eighteenth centuries. Jean-Baptiste Labat, a Dominican priest, naturalist, and botanist who undertook a series of voyages
to the French Antilles from 1694 to 1706, claimed that his trips proved
that the idea of the Greeks was false. He wrote, "We still see today that
the famous schools endorse very seriously that the Torrid Zone is uninhabitable because of the continual and excessive heat which reigns there.
This notion was pardonable before the voyages of Christopher Columbus . . . but to uphold it yet seems to me to be ridiculous and pigheaded."[31]

The division of the earth into the five zones also was a means by
which natural historians illustrated the differences among peoples, their
sexual activities, their levels of civilization, and their forms of government. According to many Enlightenment thinkers, the heat of the tropical sun intensified the sexual longings of the region's inhabitants. Because sexual activity consumed the lives of men and women in the Torrid
Zone, they had little time to ensure political freedom for themselves. Instead, they lived indolently and were subjected to the rule of cruel and
arbitrary tyrants.[32]

The most famous Enlightenment proponent of the theory that pro-
posed that environmental factors, like climate, shaped and conditioned

cultures across the globe was Charles-Louis de Secondat, Baron de Montesquieu.[33] In *The Spirit of the Laws*, Montesquieu devoted an entire section to "the laws in their relation to the nature of the climate." According to the philosopher, the heat of the Torrid Zone led to extreme physical sensitivity. The lively and excitable passions of the region's inhabitants then produced constant sexual arousal and fulfillment and other immoral behavior, including crime. Montesquieu also claimed the high temperatures of the region "can be so excessive that the body there will be absolutely without strength." As a result, the people were lazy and more subject to being enslaved because they lacked "the strength of spirit necessary to guide one's own conduct." Montesquieu also observed that differences in climates played a part in the variety of diseases that existed across the globe. Therefore, the residents of different climatic zones experienced distinct ailments.[34]

The question whether Saint Domingue was the epitome of the Torrid Zone formed an important theme in most books written about the French colony in the eighteenth century. There was a demand for European men to serve as plantation managers in place of absentee French planters, many of whom avoided Saint Domingue out of mortal fear. The colony required an influx of French women in order to bridge the uneven sex ratio that existed between men and women. European women, the commentators argued, would bring marriage, children, and stability. They would replace the female *sang-mêlés* as the women of choice for the white male residents of Saint Domingue. But what could these new arrivals expect? Wealth and long lives? Or poverty and swift deaths?

Over the course of the century, the phrase Torrid Zone, when used in reference to Saint Domingue, was a way to differentiate between climates and a means of talking about the cruel disease environment said to exist on the island. Moreau de Saint-Méry wrote, "Saint Domingue is very murderous . . . I would betray the truth, if I were to say that the scorching climate of the Torrid Zone is as favorable to the population as that of the Fortunate Zones. . . . [O]ne cannot refrain from being struck . . . by the speed with which one is attacked and beaten to the ground."[35] Physician N. Bertin also acknowledged that the climate contributed to the ill health experienced by new arrivals.[36] As late as 1803, medical practitioners were arguing for the merits of the designation. During the Haitian Revolution, Citizen Délorme maintained, "One sees that the Torrid Zone is the most deadly to its inhabitants, and . . . the birthplace of all the destructive agents of man. . . . We are led naturally to think that there is a great analogy between the diseases of different places under the same latitude."[37]

Disease in Saint Domingue could be traced to both the disease ecology of the island and the pathological effects of slavery. The murderous fevers that Europeans experienced when they first arrived in Saint Domingue reinforced the colony's reputation as the Torrid Zone. Eighteenth-century French physicians agreed that Saint Domingue was an unhealthy location for travelers from Europe. Disease had the possibility of meeting immigrants at the docks, helping them from the ship and into freshly dug graves. Physician Antoine Poissonnier-Desperrières claimed, "The French, who go to Saint Domingue . . . who had enjoyed good health during their journey, fall ill, and perish soon after landing."[38] The climate, the food, and the air one breathed all conspired to kill the newcomers.

Europeans fretted over their trips to Saint Domingue because of the dangerous diseases that stalked them there. Most of these newcomers were male, and the illness they feared most was *mal de Siam*, or yellow fever. Eighteenth-century medical writers working in Saint Domingue agreed that French immigrants to the colony had reason to be frightened of the disease. Author and royal physician Jean-Baptiste-René Pouppée-Desportes observed, "This disease attacks rather indifferently all the Europeans who are newly arrived in the Colony."[39] Malaria also posed a danger to French arrivals. Poissonnier-Desperrières observed, "New arrivals are subject to a burning fever . . . & to a particular fever, which differs in its beginning, its progress, its state, & its decline from those that reign in Europe." He added, "Climate was less dangerous to Creoles than to the French who are accustomed to temperate air, to air that is full of nourishing juices, & to a strong and continuous movement."[40] Nonetheless, Creole men, who had developed immunity to these killers, risked contracting diseases of civilization: alcoholism, gout, and heart disease. They also suffered from a variety of sexually transmitted diseases that included syphilis and gonorrhea.

Eighteenth-century physicians emphasized that the white women, both European and Creole, tended to fare better in the tropics than their male counterparts. According to the medical wisdom of the time, women fought off and survived diseases that decimated men. Nicolas Bourgeois provided evidence of this phenomenon in his travel book entitled *Voyages intéressans dans différentes colonies françaises, espagnoles, anglaises.* He noted, "The women are here the proof of the goodness of the climate: they reach a very advanced age, despite being subjected to the same sicknesses as the men."[41] Poissonnier-Desperrières likewise remarked, "All things being equal, the women run less risk than the men, the accidents with which they meet are always less grave."[42] Finally, Pouppée-Desportes observed, "The *mal de Siam* (yellow fever) struck down a countless number of men in a short period of time; but I have seen only one woman who has been attacked."[43]

According to medical practitioners in Saint Domingue, the benefits that a woman experienced in the midst of the Torrid Zone could be traced back to her unique physical makeup, most especially to the menses that she experienced. Bourgeois claimed that a woman's superior health was completely natural and resulted from her ability to purge herself. Pouppée-Desportes also attributed women's lower risk for *mal de Siam* to their monthly evacuations. Finally, Creole women enjoyed better health because of the meticulous nature of their toilet, and by not abandoning themselves to the hedonistic pleasures in which men participated.[44]

The plantations of the Caribbean were also the final earthly destinations for many slaves who suffered from smallpox, scurvy, and scabies during the voyage from Africa. J. F. Lafosse, a physician who specialized in plantation medicine, wrote, "I believe . . . that the greatest accidents come from . . . the cruel situation in which are found the unfortunates in the majority of the slaving ships. One knows that they are, so to speak, piled up one on top of the other, that the air that they respire there can only be impure and that the food that nourishes them is very dangerous because of its age and bad quality."[45] Africans received an unfamiliar and inadequate diet that was often rancid due to the lack of supplies on lengthy sea voyages. Some captives aboard slaving vessels refused to eat or were unable to eat as a result of seasickness and overcrowded and unclean conditions.[46]

The ships that dropped anchor in the ports of Saint Domingue were repositories of disease and death. Inspection and quarantine were part of the European medical tradition for more than four centuries, and Saint Domingue officials passed numerous ordinances that required physicians and surgeons to investigate the health conditions aboard recently arrived slave ships—but the profusion of laws attempting to legislate against the import of disease bears witness to the impotence of such legislation. Dreaming of the money to be made from the sale of slaves, the *capitaines négriers* (captains of the slaving vessels) hurried their human cargo, and the disease among them, from the holds of the ships onto the docks of Saint Domingue.[47] Once disembarked and before being sold, slaves were kept in storehouses in the port cities and towns of Saint Domingue. Moreau de Saint-Méry said these warehouses "offered the heart-rending spectacle of humanity disowned by greed," and were too often "the scene of cruel epidemics."[48] Fearing the outbreak of disease and moved by the needs of the slave economy, the leaders of Cap-François approved the establishment of a hospital for newly arrived slaves in 1782.[49]

About half the newly arrived slaves perished in the first three years.

Amebic dysentery was the greatest killer during this period.[50] *Nouveaux* also died from *mal d'estomach,* a disease that eighteenth-century physician Jean-Damien Chevalier described as "pain in the epigastric region, the whole body is heavy, sleep overwhelms them, in waking, in working, they always want to be lying down . . . they have a devouring hunger."[51] Scholars, however, disagree about what disease *mal d'estomach* actually was. A general wasting away, sleeping sickness, pica (consumption of inorganic matter such as clay), beriberi (vitamin B_1 deficiency), and hookworm anemia have all been mentioned as possible diagnoses. Whatever disease it may have been, nutritional deficiencies brought on by the Middle Passage and by the change in diet on the plantation likely accounted for it.[52]

Those *nouveaux* who survived the voyage from Africa and the period of acclimatization had to face the horrible living conditions of the plantations, surroundings that affected the health of all slaves whether African or Creole. Slaves generally received a weekly ration of meat or fish and cereal from the *gérant,* but the remainder of their diet was their responsibility. Planters set aside a small portion of the property where slaves were responsible for producing their own food. Slaves cultivated this soil, normally of very poor quality, during their two-hour break, which lasted from noon until two o'clock. Slaves also worked at their plots on Sundays and feast days, which were, by law, days when no plantation work could be completed by the enslaved labor force. Like many other laws, this statute often was ignored in the face of economic considerations, meaning that slaves had even less time to care for their own meager plots of land. Slaves grew a variety of foods in these gardens in order to supplement the provisions provided by the plantation managers. Manioc, sweet potatoes, millet, maize, rice, and peas were common crops (Figure 2). Slaves also fished and searched for crabs.[53]

The long workday and time spent tending their own gardens led to fatigue and the depletion of any nutritional reserves the slaves were able to establish. Slaves started their day at five o'clock in the morning, rested for a short time at midday, and continued working until daylight faded. Slaves labored longer and harder during harvest time. In addition, slaves toiled on public works ordered by the king. These *corvées* were very unpopular with planters because they further exhausted the plantation's labor force, led to *marronnage,* and resulted in disease epidemics.[54]

The clothing and houses of the slaves contributed to their poor physical state. According to law, masters had to provide slaves with two changes of clothing, or a certain length of cloth, once a year. Again, as with the ordinance on food rations, this law was usually ignored. Enslaved males made do with a shirt and pair of pants, while women wore a skirt and a

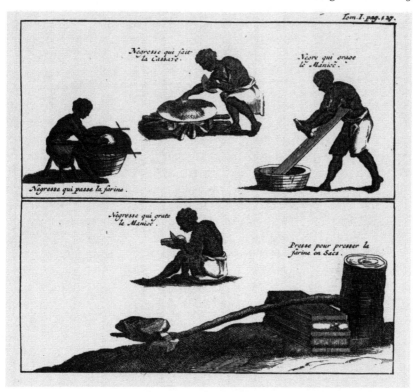

Figure 2. Enslaved man and women preparing manioc. Note the lack of adequate clothing and footwear, which posed health risks for African and Afro-Caribbean slaves. Jean-Baptiste Labat, Nouveau Voyage aux Isles de l'Amérique *(The Hague, 1724), 1: 127. Used with the permission of the Library Company of Philadelphia.*

shirt. Both men and women wore clothes made of tow, a material made from hemp. Travel book author Girod-Chantrans said that it "was not rare to see grown men and women nearly nude, or covered with rags so disgusting that they inspired both horror and pity."[55] Slave children were usually naked. The lack of footwear led to frequent wounds, which contributed to the high rate of tetanus among the slave population. As with clothing, the houses did nothing to shelter the slave from the elements. They were miserable structures without windows, and the poor wood of which they were made let in the cool night air and the heat, as well as the rain.[56]

    The overwork and lack of proper food and clothing that slaves endured played a role in the slave's inability to avoid falling prey to respiratory illnesses. Pulmonary diseases were among the most common maladies from which slaves suffered and died. Some such respiratory illnesses were bronchitis, whooping cough, pneumonia, and tuberculosis.[57]

Slaves also suffered from *maladies vermineuses* (diseases caused by intestinal worms). Slaves developed guinea worm disease after drinking water containing tiny water fleas infected by *D. medinensis*, a nematode parasite.[58] Like the guinea worm, hookworm also weakened the slave population and caused death. Slaves contracted hookworm by coming into contact with infected larvae in soil contaminated by human feces or by ingesting contaminated food. Fearing that deaths from parasites might have been the work of malicious slaves, many planters commissioned their surgeons to perform autopsies. Jean-Barthélemy Dazille, a former naval surgeon and physician who studied the medical and physical treatment of enslaved men and women, recorded that "the opening of all the cadavers of slaves, dead from ordinary illnesses, revealed the intestines stuffed with worms." The pulmonary diseases that physicians and surgeons observed in slaves were likely worsened by infections caused by the burrowing of larvae in the lungs. Medical practitioners generally recommended that slaves be given a purgative or emetic in order to force the worms from the system.[59]

Finally, slaves endured the agonies of *pian* (yaws). Considered by eighteenth-century physicians as a form of venereal disease, yaws, an endemic treponemal infection transmitted by casual contact, led to severe facial disfigurement. It also resulted in a condition known as crab yaws, so called because of the crablike way victims walked due to lesions on the soles of the feet.[60]

Saint Domingue's reputation as a breeder of disease was not confined to the colony, to its metropole, nor to the eighteenth century. Philadelphia physicians blamed French refugees from then war-torn Saint Domingue for importing yellow fever into the city and causing the epidemic of 1793. Many Philadelphia doctors agreed with William Currie's assessment that the disease came from "St. Domingo, from whence a multitude of the inhabitants fled at different times in the summer of 1793, on account of a desolating war, in consequence of the insurrection of slaves in that island, and took shelter in Philadelphia."[61] The College of Physicians of Philadelphia concurred with Currie's opinion, stating that the fever "was easily traced to some persons who was lately arrived from some of the West Indian Islands, where it was epidemical."[62]

Early twentieth-century American naval medical officers also classified Haiti as a country devastated by disease and worried that the island population was the source of worldwide syphilis. Navy doctors were concerned that American Marines, who were taking part in the U.S. occupation of Haiti, might contract syphilis as a result of sexual contact with Haitian women. The most outspoken proponent of this view was Charles S. Butler, a naval medical officer who served in Haiti from 1924 until 1927 as a sanitary engineer and eventually as director general of the Public Health Service on the island. Butler drew the mistaken conclusion that the disease common among Haitian women, yaws, could easily manifest itself as syphilis in the body of the occupying sailor or soldier.[63]

As recently as 1982, Americans were warned again of the physical danger posed by the population of Haiti. In that year, the U.S. Centers for Disease Control alerted the general public to the dangerous role that Haitians and Haitian immigrants played in the AIDS crisis.[64] The identification of Haitians as a high-risk population was widely debated in both medical and political circles.[65] Well aware of the damage that this charge brought to the Haitian people and their economy, the Haitian ambassador to the United States spoke out. In a letter to the editor of the *New England Journal of Medicine,* Fritz N. Cineas stated:

> The Republic of Haiti has suffered a severe injustice over the past year in the American press. Countless broadcast and print journalists have related stories attributing the origins of the acquired immunodeficiency syndrome (AIDS) to Haitians, without sufficient factual data to support this theory. . . . The volume of media stories relating Haitians and AIDS has cast a pall of gloom over the country, deterring potential business investors and tourists from venturing too near. . . . Haiti . . . has sufficient problems without being selected as a scapegoat for a mysterious ailment.[66]

Similarly, Dr. Ralph Greco observed that the stigma of AIDS had serious repercussions for Haitians who immigrated to the United States: "'Boat people' have been housed in makeshift prisons, and Haitians who have immigrated legally are housed in a different 'prison' in our ghettos."[67] One group of researchers concluded that the naming of Haitians as a high-risk group for AIDS may have resulted from "the surveillance of a 'captive' population of patients, such as interned Haitian refugees."[68] Many of the participants in this debate, however, failed to realize that the identification of Haitians as a high-risk population was in keeping with the historic view of Haiti as a place of disease and death.[69]

Just as the American government attempted to limit the spread of AIDS through misguided immigration policies in the 1980s, the French government in the eighteenth century tried to lessen the incidence of disease in the colony through the establishment of a massive medical bureaucracy. As we will see in chapter 2, royally appointed medical professionals, private health practitioners, and military physicians and surgeons struggled to stop disease and the deaths that accompanied it.

2 *European Medicine in the Torrid Zone*

> Are not all citizens obliged to arm themselves in order to repulse the invasion of an enemy that menaces the Republic? This enemy, Gentlemen, is disease, whose attack is perpetual and tends always to destroy society: it is up to doctors and surgeons to combat it and stop the progress of its incursion. The Sovereign has put in their hands a part of his confidence, and oppressed humanity calls out for their care.
>
> —Charles Arthaud, *Discours prononcé à l'ouverture de la première séance publique du Cercle des Philadelphes,* 1785

The charge of Charles Arthaud, royal physician and founder of the Saint Domingue scientific and medical society, to his fellow medical practitioners to take up the fight against disease reflected the Enlightenment's radical redefinition of health. According to the *philosophes,* health was the key to happiness, and without it one was unable to fulfill one's potential; one became a trial to one's friends and a burden on society. Enlightened scholars hoped that a reformed and revitalized medicine might help in the construction of a new society that was based on the conquest of disease.[1]

Saint Domingue offered a unique testing ground for the Enlightenment's new philosophy of health. Saint Domingue was a doctor's dream, or, better yet, a medical practitioner's paradise. The need for healthy bodies, both white and black, in Saint Domingue meant that medicine and its practitioners would play important roles in both the colony's development and this novel Enlightenment experiment. There was money, prestige, and status to be had not only by cultivating the rich island soil, but also by treating the diseases that flourished there.

The medical establishment in Saint Domingue experienced a problem similar to that occurring in France in the same period. The fluidity of medical roles within the traditional corporate structure led to conflicts among its branches. The colonial medical establishment also encountered difficulties that were unique to the island. The plantation economic structure gave rise to a peculiar, unlicensed, and, therefore, unlawful practitioner called the plantation surgeon, the nemesis of the educated Enlightenment practitioner. Saint Domingue's identity as an island colony also guaranteed that the official civilian medical community would compete with and enter into conflict with the military and naval medical community, most notably with naval surgeons. Medical legislation, which sought to ensure boundaries between the branches of the medical hierarchy, between licensed and unlicensed practitioners, and between civilian and military medicine, was ineffective because laws were simply disregarded or violated and enforcement was lax. Furthermore, the circumventing of public health measures ensured that disease would occur and spread quickly. As a result of these conditions, many practitioners, as we will see later in the book, turned to enslaved healers for assistance.

Medicine: Transformation and Tradition

The practice and science of medicine were undergoing drastic changes both in Europe and in Saint Domingue. One significant characteristic of medicine in the Age of Enlightenment was the development of nosology. Taking their cue from natural historians like Carolus Linnaeus, medical taxonomists classified diseases according to symptoms. They hoped that systematizing medical information might aid them in understanding the sicknesses they observed. They even dreamed that their collection and organization of medical facts might help them discover the natural laws responsible for sickness and health.[2] Physicians and other medical workers in Saint Domingue, likewise, categorized the illnesses to which the residents of the colony were susceptible and those to which they were immune. By drawing conclusions about the diseases they had classified, they expected to aid the suffering.

Eighteenth-century medical practitioners also stressed change and amelioration. The idea of the "medicable," or those patient populations to whom the medical community offered its assistance, was enlarged to include women (obstetrics) and children (pediatrics), and greater emphasis was placed on proper hygiene to prevent illness and improve life.[3] The Enlightenment's emphasis on amelioration made its way to Saint Domingue in the second half of the eighteenth century as physicians, surgeons, and colonial leaders tried to improve the physical surroundings of the colony by instituting public health measures. Many residents of Saint Domingue wanted to better the lives of enslaved men and women. Economically, one might retain more slaves, who before had died of disease brought on by neglect, overwork, and inadequate clothing and shelter. Politically, planters and proslavery advocates responded to charges brought by the abolitionists that the slaves labored and lived in inhumane circumstances. In addition, the possibility that the slave trade might be ended convinced many slaveholders to provide better care in order to keep the present population of slaves healthy and alive. This change in the care that enslaved men and women received emerged most markedly during the 1760s. France's fight for empire during this decade made slaving voyages to Africa more difficult. Fearing that the supply of African slaves would be cut off, colonists attempted to ensure the health of slaves they already owned. Proprietors also began to encourage slave women to reproduce. This emphasis on natural increase represented an important transformation in the role of slave women from laborers to reproducers.[4]

In France, the closing decades of the eighteenth century also witnessed the Revolution, an event that transformed politics, society, culture, and the practice of medicine. The old corporations or guilds were abolished in March 1791 and popular medical practitioners, such as empirics, flourished. By the early nineteenth century, French political leaders demanded that medical workers apply for certification in their chosen professions. As a result, the modern medical disciplines of pharmacy, surgery, and medicine arose and effectively created professional monopolies that excluded empirics and other medical practitioners, such as bonesetters, from mainstream modern medicine.[5] Arthaud was well aware that the political instability in France and Saint Domingue might bring about changes in medicine. Mindful of his chance to affect the future of medicine, he presented his suggestions on how to improve the practice of colonial medicine to lawmakers in France and Saint Domingue in 1791. In *Observations sur les Lois, concernant la Médecine et la Chirurgie dans la Colonie de St. Domingue* (observations on the laws, concerning medicine and surgery in the colony of Saint Domingue), Arthaud outlined the responsibilities of official medical practitioners. He also urged national and colonial legislators to recognize the medical care provided by enslaved women and females of color, work previously prohibited by law.[6]

The work of enslaved healers and the colonists who sought out, utilized, and influenced their therapies also revolutionized the practice of medicine. These men and women were true medical revolutionaries. The push to employ inoculation in the colony and in France came from the use of the technique by enslaved men and women. Likewise, medical practitioners investigated and recommended the herbal remedies of the slave healers. Finally, Afro-Caribbean slave medicine incorporated elements of Western medicine.

In spite of the changes that characterized medicine in the eighteenth century, its practitioners looked to the past for both theoretical information and practical techniques. In the first half of the eighteenth century, doctors relied overwhelmingly on humoral or Galenic medical theory to explain how and why diseases occurred. Medical tradition taught physicians and other medical practitioners that disease was caused by an imbalance of humors in the body. The humors included blood, yellow bile, black bile, and phlegm. In order to rid the body of excess humor, a physician might order his patient to be bled by a surgeon, or recommend a laxative, an emetic, or a sudorific to expel putrid matter from the body.[7]

The medical theory that most influenced the study and practice of medicine in Saint Domingue during the closing decades of the eighteenth century was environmentalism, which posited that disease was an outcome of one's environment. The climate in which one lived, the air one breathed, the water one drank, even the work one did all played roles in the development of disease. This philosophy looked to the wisdom of Hippocrates, on which many eighteenth-century medical practitioners relied to improve and advance medicine. Many colonial physicians accepted environmentalism as a result of the tremendous influence that the *Société Royale de Médecine* in Paris had on medical thought. Many colonial doctors were members and correspondents of this institution and toed its ideological line.[8]

The popularity of environmentalism as well as the miasmatic theory (which held that disease emerged from rotting vegetable matter) explains why physicians took a preventive approach to disease in Saint Domingue. Physicians harped on the importance of draining swamps and bogs, removing refuse, properly ventilating homes, and adequately burying bodies, whether animal or human. Dazille said it was the duty of medical men to suggest the proper locations for hospitals, cemeteries, butcheries, and tanneries, and that they should advise citizens on what types of building materials ensured proper health. In order to bring about widespread environmental improvements, medical practitioners realized that they needed to enlist the aid and power of the French and Saint Domingue governments. They felt confident that they would find assistance there.

Saint Domingue's Medical Bureaucracy

Much of what we know about Saint Domingue's official medical world and its efforts to improve the practice of medicine comes from the work of Arthaud, a true colonial renaissance man. Arthaud served as a royal physician and founded, presided over, and acted as secretary to and historian of the *Cercle des Philadelphes*. Despite its rather short existence, the *Cercle des Philadelphes* rivaled any French provincial academy of the time. It had a fine publishing record, established ties with its metropolitan equivalent, the *Académie Royale des Sciences* in Paris, claimed an international membership, and associated with other learned institutions, such as the American Philosophical Society in Philadelphia and several French provincial academies. The *Cercle des Philadelphes* was one of a number of colonial organizations that promoted science and medicine in the eighteenth century. Similar associations were found in the Caribbean colonies of Jamaica and Barbados. Like other colonial academies, the *Société Royale des Sciences et des Arts du Cap-François* emphasized the practical benefits of studying science and medicine. Its collection of essays on epizootic diseases and a study of *tétanos* were eagerly read by medical practitioners and laymen in Saint Domingue.[9] As leader of the *Cercle des Philadelphes*, Arthaud associated and corresponded with the leading academic societies of his day, including the American Philosophical Society, the Royal Society of Medicine of Paris, the Academy of Surgery, and the Society of the Sciences of Montpellier. In addition, he was a member of Saint Domingue's economic and social elite; he owned an estate valued at 630,000 colonial *livres* and was related to Moreau de Saint-Méry by marriage.[10] Besides writing works on smallpox, animal diseases, and the activities of the *Cercle des Philadelphes*, Arthaud provided an account of the duties expected of public and private medical workers, a partial history of medical legislation enacted in the colony, and his own suggestions on the future of colonial medicine.

THE ROYAL PRACTITIONERS

The most powerful members of Saint Domingue's official medical establishment were the royally appointed medical practitioners. The appointment of medical administrators by the Crown was not unique to Saint Domingue; royal physicians, surgeons, and other medical authorities also existed in France. In 1693 the Crown selected the first *médecin du roi*, whose duties included representing the Crown in the medical college, advising on legal cases, and performing autopsies.[11] In 1701 the Crown named a Montpellier physician, Michel Lopez de Pas, Saint Domingue's original royal physician.[12] The *médecin du roi*, or the chief medical officer in the colony, verified the degrees of newly arrived doctors, presided at the licensing exams of surgeons, apothecaries, and midwives, assessed pharmacies and the drug supplies of surgeons and apothecaries, and monitored the accounts of their fellow physicians and surgeons.[13]

Royal physicians, however, were sometimes lax in their verification of medical degrees. As a result, they gave out licensing certificates to men who had never studied physic or who did not possess practical clinical experience. They also granted aspiring doctors permission to practice without formally meeting with them and inspecting their qualifications as the story of Louis Bourdais reveals. "Doctor" Bourdais was a tailor, who stole a medical degree that had been officially registered at the *Conseil Supérieur*, and practiced both medicine and surgery for ten years. The *Conseil Supérieur* finally prohibited Bourdais from practicing medicine after a group of physicians raised a stink over his botched handling of a medical case. Eager to tear into the fabric of the human body, the former tailor had cut open an aneurism that he had mistaken for an abscess in the carotid artery of a patient's neck.[14]

Royal physicians were not only expected to supervise lesser-ranking medical workers but also were required to perform duties designed to guarantee public health and safety. In order to ensure the continued defense of his majesty's most important colony, the royal physician provided medical care to the sick confined in military hospitals and inspected these institutions. He also certified the states of health of common soldiers as well as military officers. The royal physician examined slave ships and their human cargo for contagious diseases and had the authority to quarantine vessels if the need arose. These measures were designed to guard against epidemics and their accompanying loss of both human life and economic profit. Captains of slaving ships, in a hurry to sell their cargo, disregarded the quarantines.[15]

In addition to military hospitals and slave ships, royal physicians also inspected prisons. A report on the Royal Prisons of the Cap submitted by royal physician Arthaud in 1786 provides some insight into this particular duty. Arthaud's account recorded the frightful conditions present in the part of the prison that housed slaves. Arthaud and his surgical associate noted that the latrines were defective, which resulted in the accumulation of a stagnant pool of excrement. The royal medical practitioners judged that this situation led to ill health and suggested that colonial authorities construct better sanitation facilities in order to arrest the progress of disease. These suggestions, however, bore little fruit because in a report five years later Arthaud again mentioned the existence of disease in the prisons. In this case, the victims were white prisoners, who, unlike the slaves, had no infirmary where their illnesses could be treated.[16]

Royal physicians also provided medical care at the colony's largest hospital, the *Hôpital de la Charité*, near Cap-François. The hospital housed approximately one thousand patients, including military officers, common soldiers, private patients, and the suffering poor. The hospital was self-sufficient, with kitchens, bakeries, baths, stables, a pharmacy, housing for medical staff, a botanical garden, and quarters for the hospital's slaves. The *Hôpital de la Charité* also served as a medical school for physicians, surgeons, and apothecaries from France who were required by law to serve one year at the hospital before establishing private practice in the colony.[17]

The Brothers of Charity, a Catholic religious order, were responsible for the day-to-day operation of the *Hôpital de la Charité*. The Brothers were not unique to Saint Domingue; they also served in hospitals in France, where they were singled out for their humane care of the insane and their surgical skills.[18] In the colony's largest hospital, they furnished basic nursing care and distributed food. But comments made by Arthaud indicate that the Brothers of Charity overstepped professional boundaries and provided surgical and medical care for which he felt they were not properly qualified. Arthaud wrote, "It is necessary to stamp out the pretensions of the Brothers of Charity, to strip them of their usurpations." Arthaud's antagonistic attitude toward the Brothers of Charity mirrored attacks made against the religious community by surgeons in Paris, who accused the clerics of practicing medicine and surgery without adequate training.[19]

The Crown also appointed a first *chirurgien du roi* (royal surgeon), who performed duties similar to those of the first royal physician. The royal surgeon presided over surgical matters such as the licensing of newly arrived surgeons. Following the traditional corporate structure of medicine, the powers of the first royal surgeon were subsumed under those of the *médecin du roi*. Thus, he acted as a subordinate to the royal physician and worked alongside the doctor treating soldiers and sailors; visiting and inspecting slave ships, poorhouses, hospitals, and plantations; assisting at the licensing examinations of apothecaries and midwives; and offering medical reports to the colonial administration.[20]

The Crown also designated chief health officers in other areas of colonial medicine. The royal apothecary, along with the royal physician and surgeon, inspected medical supplies aboard ship and those belonging to surgeons. The royal obstetrician-physician offered midwifery courses and licensed midwives, while the royally sanctioned veterinarian inspected plantations devastated by animal disease.[21]

The official burdens assumed by the royal medical practitioners, however, were not compensated as royally as one might suspect. By the end of the Old Regime, royal physicians earned lower annual salaries than plantation surgeons, many of whom never had received formal or adequate medical training. A top-ranking physician appointed by the Crown received 2,400 colonial *livres* for a year's work compared to the annual salary of a plantation surgeon, which averaged about 4,000 colonial *livres*. A *chirurgien du roi* could expect even less; his salary was a mere 1,800 colonial *livres*.[22] The royal physician and surgeon, however, received special benefits and exemptions that contributed nicely to their total annual incomes. The *médecin du roi* was exempt from paying taxes on twelve of the slaves that he owned. Both royal medical administrators also earned fees when they supervised at licensing exams. In addition, they augmented their official salaries by combining several medical posts within the administration and by their earnings made in private practice. The *chirurgien du roi*, for instance, made money by treating prisoners, including the slaves forced to work on chain gangs, and at other times by serving as a surgeon on a plantation.[23]

PRACTITIONERS AND PRIVATE PRACTICE

Physicians, surgeons, apothecaries, midwives, and veterinarians in private practice worked in Saint Domingue. Tradition dictated that physicians stood at the top of the medical hierarchy because their work relied upon intellectual ability and book learning. They were considered the scholars of the medical world as a result of their university education, which included a master of arts degree, four years of medical study, the receipt of the doctorate, and the successful completion of a licensing examination.[24] In order to practice in Saint Domingue, physicians also were required to furnish their university credentials or their *brevets*, royal warrants that attested to their standing as physicians, to the colonial administrators and the first royal physician.

Like his counterpart in France, a physician in Saint Domingue generally lived in an urban area, whether a coastal city or a large town in the colony's interior. Economically and socially colonial physicians, like French doctors, were members of the middle class.[25] Over the course of the eighteenth century, some high-ranking physicians in Saint Domingue came to be recognized as *grands blancs*. Medical practice definitely offered the chance of a more lucrative lifestyle and was a unique position within the colony. Out of a population of approximately 500,000, only 26 men claimed the title of doctor in 1791.[26]

Physicians treated a varied clientele. A doctor might tend to a sailor suffering from venereal disease in the morning, then, later in the day, visit an important French bureaucrat, who also endured venereal disease as well as gout. Slaves and free men and women of mixed race had access to Saint Domingue physicians and appear in their records. Pouppée-Desportes reported that he treated an enslaved cook who complained of pain in the upper right portion of the abdomen, or the area of the liver. Pouppée-Desportes advised the master to move the slave to another part of the household, but the master refused. The royal physician may have suggested this move because a different occupation may have been a little less fatiguing. But because the enslaved man was a cook, and, therefore, a talented and trained member of the plantation household, the master felt compelled to keep him at his post. The cook's condition deteriorated to such an extent that the slave man himself sought out Pouppée-Desportes for assistance. The physician noted that the man had lost weight and that his liver felt firm to the touch. Pouppée-Desportes prescribed bloodletting, an *infusion apéritive* (a tea to stimulate the man's appetite), and a poultice, or a soft mixture usually heated and spread on a cloth that is then applied to the affected area. Three months later, the man's condition had not improved, and his lower extremities became swollen with fluid. Pouppée-Desportes ordered the man to be scarified, or cut superficially, to evacuate the excess liquid from his body. The cook eventually died, and Pouppée-Desportes conducted an autopsy. He found the abdomen filled with three to four pints of "water" and signs of liver disease, the diagnosis Pouppée-Desportes eventually applied to the man's condition.[27]

Surgeons ranked below physicians like Pouppée-Desportes in the traditional medical hierarchy because surgery was a manual occupation, a trade that depended on mechanical skill, not intellectual theorizing. Unlike university-trained physicians, surgeons generally were taught by means of an apprentice system. When an apprentice finished his period of service, his master awarded him a certificate that testified he had completed his training.[28] An example of such a certificate is that of Pierre Didier, a Saint Domingue surgeon who fled the colony at the start of the revolution (Figure 3). He arrived in the United States in 1794, settled in Delaware, and served as a physician to the Dupont family and its employees from 1802 until his death in 1830.[29]

Surgical practitioners performed a wide variety of procedures, but bloodletting was the most common service they provided, usually under orders from a physician. In the eighteenth century, bloodletting was not

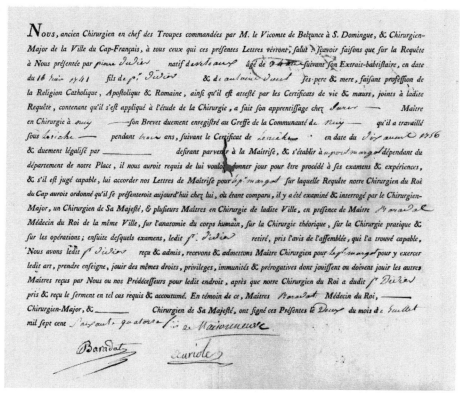

Figure 3. Certificate to practice surgery presented to Pierre Didier on 2 July 1774 by Monsieur Baradat. Winterthur Manuscripts, Group 10, Series A, DuPont Family Miscellany. Courtesy of the Hagley Museum and Library.

only a means of fighting illness, but also a way to prevent sickness in the first place. Physicians even encouraged newly arrived Europeans to be bled before disembarking ship to prevent the onset of fever.[30] Yet by the closing decades of the eighteenth century, some physicians and surgeons avoided drastic bloodletting. By that time, they advocated a more cautious therapy, called expectant therapeutics, which enjoyed favor both in Saint Domingue and elsewhere. Proponents of this new medical care began with mild remedies and allowed nature to take its course.[31] Surgeons made up the largest segment of the Saint Domingue medical community. Unlike physicians, surgeons ventured outside urban areas into the countryside and onto plantations.[32] Because they outnumbered physicians, surgeons were the medical practitioners of choice for most residents of Saint Domingue. Surgeons treated members of the planter class as well as the lowliest slave. The power of the surgeons in both France and Saint Domingue was due neither to numbers alone nor to patient choice. In the age of Enlightenment, when medicine came to be viewed as a practical science, surgery enjoyed prestige as a useful art because of the development of successful surgical techniques, most notably lithotomy, or the extraction of bladder stones. Physic, on the other hand, is said to have stagnated during the eighteenth century. It relied on heroic medical therapeutics, such as purgation, in order to treat acute cases of illness. Physicians offered the same remedies but in a milder form to chronic patients, who also were put on bland diets that included herbal tisanes and white meat bouillons. Therapeutics in the eighteenth century was, as historians Laurence Brockliss and Colin Jones described it, "a science still to be forged."[33]

In France and Saint Domingue, surgeons amassed power at the expense of physicians, apothecaries, and midwives. In order to maintain the corporate distinction between physicians and surgeons and to minimize the erosion of the physician's power, a series of royal edicts appeared in Saint Domingue that attempted to control the behavior of surgeons. Doctors in France were waging a similar battle by going to court to maintain their place of superiority in the French medical establishment.[34] In Saint Domingue, laws prohibited surgeons from practicing internal medicine, the province of physicians. In addition, after 1739, colonial surgeons had to take up residency in a colonial hospital for one year and were made to attend seminars offered by the first royal physician before being allowed to practice their craft.[35]

Conflict between the top two tiers of the corporate medical structure was heated. Saint Domingue physicians lashed out at surgeons by asserting that they were ignorant providers of dangerous treatments. Pouppée-Desportes recounted an instance of surgical incompetence, saying, "The surgeon cared for the patient by following a method totally opposed to that counseled by his colleague . . . the patient was the victim [of jealousy]. . . . [H]e died three or four days later."[36] Chevalier, likewise, remarked that the ill tended to perish at the hands of surgeons and other incompetent practitioners of the medical arts.[37]

Surgeons not only encroached on areas of medicine normally reserved for physicians, but also infiltrated the practice of midwifery. Experienced midwives had trained young women in the art, but the status and authority of midwives deteriorated and gave way to the power of the educated physician and his surgical associate. In Saint Domingue, surgeons trained local midwives, who then received their licenses after being examined by a board of physicians and authorized midwives.

Both surgeons and female midwives cared for pregnant women, delivered infants, and tended to the needs of mothers and children. They were well aware of medical legislation that affected their work. They knew of the 1725 law that required all deliveries undertaken by a midwife to be witnessed by a master of surgery, who would assume control of the situation if a difficult birth presented itself.[38] In 1765 a law was passed prohibiting female midwives and surgeons from delivering in secret any baby without alerting the colonial authorities.[39] This decree may have been designed to guard against acts of infanticide committed after pregnancies had been concealed.

The power of the state not only extended to licensing and deliveries but also dictated the amount of money midwives made. Midwives in Saint Domingue anticipated set fees for the infants they delivered after a 1757 colonial declaration specified types of deliveries and the fee chargeable for each. Reflecting the racial divisions within the colony, fees depended upon whether the mother was free or enslaved. In addition, problematic births paid more than natural ones. Deliveries in cities or towns had lower fees than those in the countryside; moreover, the midwife received extra pay for the time her trip took. Fees ranged from 15 to 120 colonial *livres,* and in addition midwives got food rations from military storehouses for themselves, their spouses, their children, and their servants.[40]

A third group with whom physicians and surgeons quarreled was the apothecaries, who occupied the third rung on the traditional corporate ladder and who were considered superior to female midwives. The role of the apothecary was to prepare and dispense medications prescribed by a physician. The arrival of the apothecary trade occurred rather late in Saint Domingue, when it emerged as a specialization growing out of the surgical trade in 1764. This unique evolution explains in part why surgeons in Saint Domingue, unlike those in France, enjoyed the right to use drugs in their practice.[41]

Apothecaries tended to live in urban areas in order to be near the physicians on whom their livelihood depended. They also likely resided in coastal cities to have access to the ships that carried patent medicines from France. An announcement of the sale of a drugstore in the *Gazette de Saint Domingue,* the colony's most important newspaper, reveals how important commerce with France was to the drug trade. MM. Escavy and Company, a family-run operation composed of druggists and apothecaries, reassured the public that, despite its takeover of Sieur Aubin's drugstore, it would continue to supply quality pharmaceutical products gained from its business with Marseille drug wholesalers.[42] Apothecaries made up only a small part of the Saint Domingue medical establishment; by 1791 the colony claimed only 24 of them.[43]

Like other members of the medical establishment, apothecaries had to submit to licensing exams headed by a board of physicians, surgeons, and fellow apothecaries before being allowed to open a shop or engage in the drug trade. Fears over widespread poisoning undertaken by slaves led to the strict regulation of pharmacy. A 7 February 1738 law, for example, prohibited surgeons, apothecaries, and druggists from entrusting to their slaves any poisons, drugs, or other compositions.[44] But Michel-René Hilliard d'Auberteuil, author of a book on Saint Domingue and its culture, recorded an incident during which a slave, and not his master, was punished for breaking this law. Hilliard d'Auberteuil noted that in 1774 a surgeon gave a packet of arsenic to his slave assistant. The arsenic eventually ended up in the pocket of another young slave who said he had received it from the surgeon's slave. Instead of punishing the surgeon as the 1738 law provided, legal authorities imprisoned the slave assistant whom Hilliard d'Auberteuil identified as a *nègre pharmacien* (slave pharmacist). The slave died in prison before a judgment could be made on his case. Hilliard thought this was a tragic incident and believed that "the imprudence of the master must . . . be punished more severely than the crime of the slave."[45]

As Hilliard's report shows, medical legislation on drug sales was rarely or properly enforced. Apothecaries and other medical practitioners simply refused to abide by them. Thus, the government enacted more prohibitions like the 1772 law forbidding apothecaries, surgeons, druggists, and captains of trading vessels from selling rat poisons composed of arsenic. The most involved law to stop suspected poisonings was the 1780 ordinance of MM. de Reynaus and le Brasseur, which restricted the sale of certain drugs and poisons, like arsenic, orpiment, and mercury chloride, solely to the *apothicaires du roi* (royal apothecaries), required these items be kept under lock and key, obliged royal apothecaries to sell these items only to doctors and surgeons, and called for records to be made of the sale and movement of toxins.[46]

Drug sellers not only faced strict regulation of their trade but also endured severe criticism by their fellow medical practitioners and lay writers. The accusation of selling tainted material was constantly leveled against pharmacists. Medicines often were outdated from lengthy sea voyages or had lost their potency because they had grown old in the shop of the druggist. Instead of formulating their own concoctions from the vegetables and minerals of the islands, the surgeons and apothecaries bought drugs from sea merchants.[47]

Saint Domingue also was home to a small number of veterinarians, whose story will be told in chapter 5. Medical workers who focused on a particular part of the human anatomy or provided services to alleviate certain medical conditions also practiced in Saint Domingue. Expert dentists, a trussmaker, and a bandager all worked in Cap-François in 1789.[48] Moreau de Saint-Méry observed that the two dentists who practiced in Cap-François were busy despite the fact that "teeth are naturally well-formed in Saint Domingue."[49]

Military Medicine and Malpractice

Saint Domingue medicine was divided into private and public practitioners as well as licensed and unlicensed medical workers. A third medical community also existed in Saint Domingue: the military medical establishment. Military medical workers were familiar sights in Saint Domingue. Army surgeons cared for soldiers who made up the regiments stationed in Port-au-Prince and Cap-François. They tended to artillery units, the militia, and admiralty officers. Likewise, naval surgeons traveled to the colony aboard the ships of the royal navy.[50]

Royally appointed medical officials in the civilian medical establishment reacted more positively to the army surgeons by allowing them to engage in private practice. Naval medical personnel, on the other hand, experienced a lukewarm reception because they were so numerous and because their medical skills were quite poor.[51] Pouppée-Desportes expressed pity for the sailors treated by these surgeons. He said the surgeons performed "frequent and abundant bloodletting . . . having no other method, than what is used in France, for illnesses of which they know nothing."[52] Whenever it appeared as if the official medical establishment was in danger of losing some of its power, its leading members made reference to the unique diseases at work in Saint Domingue. Disease became a rallying cry for high-ranking medical officials; only they had the power to deal with these ailments. The "inability" of naval surgeons to handle colonial illnesses convinced local medical authorities to pass laws forcing naval surgeons to submit to internships and examinations before they were licensed. The civilian practitioners feared that the sheer number and power of the naval medical crew threatened their professional power and independence. They took steps to restrain the naval surgeons by allowing them to treat only sailors and their families. Likewise, the naval medical authority came under the authority of the civilian government in the person of the colony's *intendant.*[53] But Bourgeois pointed out that the enforcement of these laws was not very strict. After deserting from the navy, many naval surgeons practiced without a license. Bourgeois concluded that it was the public, fooled by these illegal practitioners, who suffered the most harm.[54]

Despite the creation of a massive official medical establishment, disease remained a problem in Saint Domingue. The Enlightenment dream of a world where physicians, surgeons, and other medical practitioners conquered disease seemed as unattainable in France's most important colony as in the powerful French metropole. There were a number of reasons for this phenomenon. Although there were laws for practically every aspect of Saint Domingue life, especially ones that attempted to define appropriate medical roles and halt the spread of disease, the decrees were not enforced, and disease flourished. Police corruption was a main reason for the lax enforcement policy. A bribe could easily convince a member of the maréchaussée to turn his eyes away when, for example, a captain of a slaving vessel disembarked his wares before they were properly inspected for signs of disease. The blatant unwillingness of royal medical practitioners to perform the legal duties expected of them is another reason that medical legislation in Saint Domingue proved futile.[55]

As we have seen, medical practitioners themselves were well aware of the incompetence, lack of training, and shoddy treatment on the part of many within their ranks. Improper therapy and outdated, ineffective drugs, for instance, did nothing to stem death by disease. Such professional malpractice may have, in fact, sped the demise of ailing men and women. Medical practitioners also ineffectively battled the physical ravages created by the pathological system of slavery. The medical knowledge of the day was not equipped to deal with these sicknesses.

As we will see, laymen and laywomen as well as medical practitioners looked outside the confines of the official European medical establishment for assistance in conquering disease. Discouraged by the medical care they received from European medical workers, whites and free and enslaved people of color searched beyond the legal colonial medical community for relief. There they found a network of enslaved healers, to whose story we now turn.

3 Enslaved Healers on the Plantation

For Sale: A *Mulâtresse*, Creole, excellent subject, approximately 23 years old, good housekeeper, seamstress, excellent *hospitalière*, knows how to bleed.

—Dasylva, Duliepvre and Company, Merchants, 1781, from *Affiches Américaines*

Enslaved women on the plantations of Saint Domingue had little opportunity to gain positions of power within the slave hierarchy. By and large, women completed arduous field labor; men, on the other hand, had the chance to take up skilled positions, which provided greater material benefit, more freedom of movement, and more prestige. The work performed by female enslaved healers is an exception to this century-long colonial trend. Both masters and slaves perceived *hospitalières, infirmières,* and midwives as significant members of the slave hierarchy. Plantation managers and their employers exploited them for economic gain and highlighted their medical work to combat abolitionist attacks. At the same time, these women healers, like *commandeurs,* were leaders of the slave community, privileged members of the slave hierarchy, and significant participants in slave resistance and rebellion.

Plantation work was divided according to gender. Women dominated field labor; they prepared the soil, weeded, and cut sugar cane. Female slaves were members of the three fieldwork gangs: the first work gang, which completed the most difficult labor; the second work gang, which was composed of expectant and nursing mothers, newly arrived slaves, and the less physically fit and which was responsible for weeding; and the third work gang, which was made up of children between the ages of eight and thirteen and which did small tasks such as removing cane trash. Women were relegated to the fields because females did the majority of agricultural work in the parts of West Africa from where women and men were taken. The physical strength ascribed to female slaves, which assumed animal-like dimensions, also justified the backbreaking labor to which they were subjected. In the minds of the French, the African woman and her Creole descendants were nothing more than beasts of burden.[1]

Besides laboring in the fields, female slaves fed the sugar mills, an extremely dangerous task because of the chance of getting caught in the fast-moving rollers. Women lost fingers, limbs, and their lives placing cane in the mills. The association between mill feeding and women was so great that male slaves considered it a punishment and a dishonor to be assigned to the task. Planters designated women as laborers in the distillation of local rum as well.[2]

Women acted as peddlers too. They sold excess produce from their own garden plots, chickens they raised, small handmade items, and herbs. Some peddlers were so adept that their masters appointed them as hucksters who sold fruits and vegetables and whose profits reverted back to the slaveowners.[3]

Although men joined women in the fields, they had greater occasion to serve as skilled workers. Male slaves labored as coopers, boiler men, and teamsters. Within the master's household, enslaved men worked as cooks, valets, and coachmen. Women too occupied skilled positions; they served as housekeepers, seamstresses, and washerwomen. The majority of enslaved women, however, made up the ranks of the unskilled plantation laborers, a fact that led historian David Geggus to conclude, "Females had much less access than their male counterparts to positions of independence, skill, and prestige."[4] The positions occupied by the *hospitalières*, *infirmières*, and midwives were significant and rather unique opportunities for women to gain power on the plantations. Thus, the story of the enslaved healers on the plantations not only contributes to an understanding of their work and the role they played in resistance and rebellion, but also enlarges our knowledge of women of power in the slave societies of the New World.

The Hospitalière

The *hospitalière* was a type of enslaved healer crucial to the healthy functioning of the plantation economy. As the gender of the noun indicates, *hospitalières* were generally women, although male slaves also are known to have served as hospital caretakers.[5] They were high-ranking slaves, occupying a place below that of *commandeurs*. Because of the important services she provided to the plantation, the *hospitalière* was a highly valuable slave; the *hospitalière* on the Hecquet Duval plantation was worth more than 3,300 colonial *livres*. As a result of her status, value, and the important services she provided to the master's slaves, the *hospitalière* was given better food and clothing—normally garments cast off by the mistress of the plantation. On the Foäche plantation, the owner instructed the plantation manager to reward the *hospitalière* with Indian petticoats. A *hospitalière* ate her meals near the main kitchen of the plantation and lived in a house that was different from those of ordinary field slaves, sometimes in the plantation hospital itself.[6]

Because of her prominent place in the slave hierarchy, the choice of a *hospitalière* was a decision not to be taken lightly. Planters as well as their managers searched for a *hospitalière* who was in good health and well-behaved. A slave woman who had been a cook or baker was also desirable because she then might be familiar with herbs and herbal remedies.[7] Père Labat suggested that planters employ a *hospitalière* who was a "wise and intelligent *Négresse*, who serves diligently . . . who keeps the beds and the infirmary clean, and who allows to enter only that which the surgeon has permitted."[8] Laborie wrote respectfully of a beloved *hospitalière*: "Long experience, with the practical knowledge of simples, have set some of those women, in many respects, above surgeons too frequently met with in the mountains. I had one, the loss of whom I shall regret all my life." He ended by saying that he was "aided by the labours of my intelligent and faithful Mari-Anna."[9]

Testimony from the eighteenth century, however, provides examples that stray far from the attributes most desired by planters and their plantation supervisors. Political commentator and slavery advocate Michel Descourtilz portrayed the *hospitalière* as "an old, feeble slave woman, often incapable of caring for herself, who is given charge of this work (at the hospital) after having been judged useless for any other type of occupation." Descourtilz's comment, however, was not a sweeping indictment of slave women who ministered to the needs of their fellow slaves, but indicated his contempt for geographically and socially isolated large-scale planters who emphasized profit over the welfare of their slaves. Descourtilz championed the proprietors of smaller plantations who constructed "hospitals where the slaves are cared for during times of illness with great attention."[10] Dazille also spoke negatively about some *hospitalières*, who he said associated themselves with desperate slaves and plotted the destruction of their fellow bondsmen and women, the master's herds, and the master himself.[11]

It is interesting that Dazille had earlier recommended to the French ministry that each large plantation construct a hospital for ailing slaves. Dazille saw the hospital as a sound economic investment. He rejected arguments that slave hospitals were simply economic drains on the plantation coffers. He reasoned that "the conservation of twenty, thirty, forty, and even fifty slaves otherwise lost each year makes up for one's financial loss." Dazille suggested that planters absorb the costs of providing better food and clothing for the slaves in order to prevent illness caused by physical neglect.[12] His advice should not be viewed as an endorsement of enslaved healers. Dazille distrusted *hospitalières* and leveled brutal attacks on other practitioners of color, including herbalists and midwives. Dazille's dislike for enslaved healers appears to have stemmed from his desire to bring the medical worlds of Saint Domingue, both official and unlicensed, under the control of the French Ministry of the Navy, the institution sponsoring his research and waging war against the civilian medical establishment in Saint Domingue.[13]

Dazille's recommendations bore legislative fruit in 1784 when each planter was obligated to establish a hospital for his or her slaves.[14] The law's ultimate aim was to maintain the current slave population and to encourage natural increase, instead of relying on high-priced slaves imported from Africa. One of the leading authorities on plantation medicine, Lafosse hoped that, by properly managing these slave hospitals, "it is really possible to augment the population on a plantation, and to prevent the numerous deaths that one observes on some plantations."[15]

Colonists also sought to better conditions among their slaves in order to combat abolitionist attacks. Not only were planters required to construct hospitals, but they were also required to provide adequate clothing, food, and free time. In order to eliminate the neglect caused by planter absenteeism, managers had to submit more precise accounts to their employers, including records of the amount and types of work performed by slaves.[16] They also were encouraged to visit the plantation hospitals daily in order to monitor the sick and the treatment prescribed.[17] Although planters and physicians in Saint Domingue sought to better the conditions under which slaves labored and lived in order to defend themselves from abolitionists, they still responded to attacks with bitterness and derision. Lafosse, for example, argued that the philosophers who rise up against slavery would make better use of their time by indicating "ways by which one is able to mitigate the harshness [of slavery], since it is for the most powerful political reasons that it seems to perpetuate itself."[18] He recognized that the immense profits that resulted from the labor of enslaved men and women contributed to the power and prestige of France.

Hospital Design

Despite the high rate of planter absenteeism, many planters took an active interest in the design and construction of the hospitals. The hospital was so important to Laborie that he included a plan of a hospital in his manual on how to effectively establish and run a coffee plantation (Figure 4).[19] Habitants heeded the advice of their fellow planters and their physicians like Lafosse, who counseled that "it will be necessary that it be isolated, far from all stagnant or marshy water, and situated on a terrain naturally drained or able to be drained. . . . It is necessary that it be paved and that the beds be elevated so that the air is able to circulate more freely, and so that it will be easier to wash and sweep the interior."[20] As a result of recommendations like those of Lafosse, the hospital was generally placed away from the slave quarters. Poles formed the basic frame of the hospital, and walls covered with a mixture of earth or quicklime and sand sheltered the occupants. The hospital usually contained three rooms: a central chamber that housed the medicine chest, fireplace, bath, and the *hospitalière's* bed, a room to one side for male patients, and a room for female patients. Slaves slept on cots or on elevated planks fixed into the walls.[21] Some planters also ordered that patients be separated according to the maladies from which they suffered; others stressed the need for adequate ventilation. After 1770 planters enlarged the hospitals by adding balconies on which slaves walked for fresh air and sun. The balconies were not only a reaction to the miasmatic theory but also represented greater control over slave patients who previously took walks in the savannas surrounding the plantation. Some plantation managers maintained discipline over sick slaves by attaching bars to the windows and chaining the slave to the bed. Plantation employees used these tools to persuade men and women who they believed faked illness to despise their hospital stays. While noting the disciplinary function of iron bars fixed to beds, Laborie also mentioned that these instruments "with their padlocks and rings" were employed "to confine those with sore legs."[22] In addition to using restraints to discourage malingering, some planters made hospital stays as disagreeable as possible. Laborie wrote, "A negroe presents himself in the morning, especially on Mondays: '*Sir, I am sick*"; his eye is clear, his tongue clean, his skin cool, and his belly soft. It is ten to one but he pretends illness. . . . [L]et him go to the hospital; take away the pipe; put

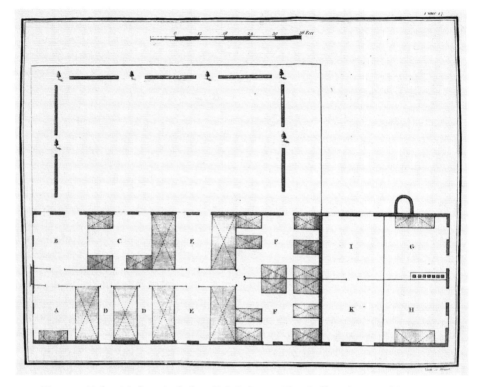

Figure 4. Laborie's hospital plan. P. J. Laborie, The Coffee Planter of Saint Domingue *(London, 1798), 94 and Plate 17. Courtesy the Newberry Library, Chicago.*

him upon a low diet, with plenty of water and clisters [i.e., clysters: enemas]; and he will be glad to be dismissed after two or three days."[23] Because of these devices and regimens, many enslaved men and women avoided being sent to the hospital because it was for them an institution of correction, not a place to recuperate from their illnesses.[24]

Plantation Surgeon

The *hospitalière* received instructions on how to care for the slaves from a plantation surgeon, the plantation manager, or the planter. Plantation medicine was by far the most lucrative area of medical practice in Saint Domingue, and many adventuresome youths traveled to the colony to take part in the surgical trade. Labat described Saint Domingue as "a true Peru for them." Labat meant that the colony was where surgeons could make a fortune. He explained, "Since the majority of them are ignorant to the utmost degree, they earn all that pleases them; and since it pleases them to earn very much, one may believe that they are soon very rich."[25] Bourgeois aptly expressed this thirst for riches when he stated, "The love of gain seduces the young men to come here to exercise medicine and surgery."[26] Plantation surgeons could make up to 8,000 colonial *livres*, much more than top-ranking physicians appointed by the Crown.[27]

Correspondence between plantation managers and their employers reveals the important functions that the plantation surgeon performed and how he was compensated for his efforts. LeCesne, a manager who oversaw a plantation belonging to the Comtes Vaudreuil and Duras, praised the efforts of the plantation surgeon, saying, "I am satisfied with Monsieur Danger, your surgeon. . . . I attribute the recovery of many of your slaves attacked by dangerous illnesses to him, his zeal, and his care." Despite being strapped with a name that would not necessarily mark him as a capable practitioner of the healing arts, Danger was a respected employee. Danger's main responsibility was to care for the slaves housed in the plantation hospital. His patients included the sick, the elderly, the disabled, and the pregnant slaves. Danger's employers rewarded him with a salary of 4,000 colonial *livres*.[28]

Plantation surgeons not only treated a wide variety of human patients but also turned their attention to animals when a qualified veterinarian was unavailable. LeCesne, for instance, depended on Danger during animal epidemics. When illness devastated the plantation's mule population, Danger performed surgery on the creatures and recommended treatments that LeCesne might use to prevent additional loss of animal life.[29]

Danger also performed autopsies, a practice common in Saint Domingue. LeCesne related Danger's dissection of a young slave woman named Rosine in one of his letters. LeCesne remarked that the slave woman had been a very capable worker who had died suddenly. The manager asked Danger to perform an autopsy to rule out the possibility that Rosine had been poisoned. The opening of her body instead revealed that the slave died from complications caused by an ectopic pregnancy. LeCesne said the fetus, aged two months, was well formed, and that Danger had preserved it in wine solution. LeCesne even offered to send it to the counts if they considered themselves amateurs in natural history.[30]

Plantation surgeons also supervised at the delivery of babies. Danger may have been summoned by LeCesne to assist the slave midwife, Brigitte, with a difficult birth. He reported the number of pregnant slaves to LeCesne, who in turn relayed this information to his employers. Suspicious that these women might procure abortions from the slave midwife, the manager kept a watchful eye on the female slaves. He also housed them in a special lying-in hospital built on the plantation when their condition had progressed.[31]

LeCesne's positive relationship and experience with Monsieur Danger differed from the negative encounters that Laborie had with plantation surgeons. One reason for this difference was the fact that Laborie ran a coffee plantation in a mountainous area, while LeCesne had charge of a sugar plantation. Laborie's land holdings and the size of his slave force may not have been as large as LeCesne's. Laborie reported, "I became tired of those mountain surgeons, who frequently could not be found at the time they were wanted; and, who, in general, are equally destitute of capacity and zeal."[32] Laborie's attitude toward the surgeons was similar to the outlook held by official colonial medical practitioners. His distaste for them led him to emphasize that planters must possess the skill to deal with medical complaints. Laborie practiced domestic medicine; by reading medical how-to books and through practical experience, he treated his own slaves and advised the *hospitalière*. He wrote, "I learned to bleed with very little trouble; and, by the help of Doctor Buchan's *Domestic Medicine*, a work which I cannot too earnestly recommend to the planters. I performed the office of physician to my sick negroes."[33] He urged his fellow planters and their employees to keep a small quantity of drugs, a balance, and a mortar on hand with which to make and dispense remedies. Despite his disdain for plantation surgeons, he admitted, "They are always necessary for luxations, fractures, and other manual operations."[34] As they made their way from plantation to plantation, the surgeons brought with them drugs and surgical instruments. Slaves who knew how to perform procedures like bloodletting and how to produce fine surgical tools also may have accompanied the plantation surgeons.[35] Even with these assistants, the plantation surgeons depended most of all on the *hospitalières.*

Hospital Practice

Whether supervised by a plantation surgeon, the plantation manager, or the planter, the daily administration of the hospital remained primarily the duty of the *hospitalière*. Planters hoped that *hospitalières* would be resolute enough to make patients follow the regime prescribed by the surgeon.[36] She performed many tasks, including dressing wounds, preparing food, and providing prescribed treatment. Chevalier wrote:

> I have seen on a *Négresse* of Monsieur Larange, our general, a small hole in the large angle of the eye, that for a long time I took as a lachrymal fistu-

lae (hole in the tear duct) because out of it came water and sometimes a little pus. Having been obliged to make a rather long voyage, at my return I demanded news of the *Négresse:* the *hospitalière* told me a Guinea worm had left by the cheek. . . . I saw the so-called fistulae healed.[37]

This *hospitalière* realized the slave woman was infested with worms and knew that a safe remedy was to allow the worm to exit the skin of its own accord without breaking or severing the worm.[38] S. J. Ducoeur-joly, a resident of Saint Domingue for more than twenty years, reported that *hospitalières* not only knew proper means of extracting Guinea worm, but also possessed methods for treating other types of worm infestation. He related that an enslaved woman demonstrated a remedy that combined lemon juice with ashes. After drinking the concoction, the ailing man recovered. Ducoeurjoly reasoned that the concoction had destroyed the worm. The remedy concluded with the prescription of several purgatives.[39] The *hospitalière* also had to know how to prepare simple remedies and how to care for minor diseases without the assistance of the surgeon. Every Sunday, she was responsible for examining the feet of her fellow slaves and removing chiggers or redbugs, parasites that caused severe itching and served as a vector for infectious diseases. Some *hospitalières* practiced other types of surgical procedures, like bloodletting.[40] Finally, *hospitalières* served as supply clerks, making sure the hospitals were stocked with linen, bandages, and dressings.[41]

The plantation records of the Counts Duras and Vaudreuil provide a glimpse into the administration of a plantation hospital. Plantation manager LeCesne furnished very detailed information about this plantation on the Cul-de-Sac plain in south central Saint Domingue, an area that led the colony in agricultural production and was an ideal location for sugar cultivation.[42] LeCesne's records indicate that Duras and Vaudreuil owned three *hospitalières*, Marie Michelle, Zabeth, and Marie Louise Vermandois, who were responsible for the health needs of approximately 400 slaves. Plantations that had more than 100 slaves generally had two or more *hospitalières*. Slave lists indicate that one woman normally outranked the others in age and in level of medical expertise.[43] In 1791 Marie Michelle was a fifty-year-old Creole slave who carried the title of *première,* or first, *hospitalière.* Second *hospitalière* Zabeth was a forty-four-year-old Creole woman and Marie Louise Vermandois, the *troisième* (third) *hospitalière* was the youngest (age 31) of the three Creole slave women. A forty-year-old Creole midwife named Brigitte assisted the three women.[44]

LeCesne's recordkeeping included precise summaries of the day-to-day administration of the plantation, which he sent to his employers every month. His records note how the slaves were employed, the amount of sugar and its by-products they produced, how many slaves were born or died, and other observations (such as the amount of rain) that LeCesne deemed significant. An important subheading under the various occupations held by the slaves is *à l' hôpital*, a term that denoted the number of slaves admitted to the plantation hospital.

LeCesne's account for the month of June 1791 shows that the hospital housed an average of thirty patients per day. The prognoses and deaths of certain patients, for example, an elderly slave man named Barba, who died at the age of 71 from *hydropisie,* or dropsy, are recorded. The *hospitalières* also treated two young slave children named Pierre-Charles and Vincent, who succumbed to *flux de sang* (literally, a bloody flow), a term that indicated the children were suffering from fever and dysentery. The *hospitalières,* likewise, ministered to a young man, Mercure, who suffered from *tétanos.* LeCesne unhappily reported that there appeared to be little hope of a recovery for Mercure. The manager hinted that the *hospitalières* were responsible for the care of the aged and infirm, two of whom were near death, an event LeCesne welcomed stating that "these losses are nothing for our plantation; the greatest misfortune for me is that the elderly outnumber the dead."[45]

Besides managing the plantation hospital, the *hospitalière* had to care for slaves segregated in the yaws (*pian*) hut. An alarming number of enslaved men and women suffered from yaws, and a variety of therapies were employed to ease their suffering. The yaws hut was normally placed away from the hospital in an area that was well ventilated like the hospital.[46] Bertin, who wrote a book on disease in the French Antilles, described the yaws hut as "a little place, . . . where the colonists lock up the *Nègres pianistes* [slaves stricken with yaws], as well as those infected with smallpox, along with one or two *Négresses* to serve them."[47] Bertin reported that the *hospitalières* rubbed a mercury-based lotion on the slaves over a six-week period and then served them a sudorific (sweat-producing) tea. This treatment reflected the humoral theory of disease. The perspiration released as a result of the mercury was believed to eliminate the harmful excess humor that had brought on the disease. Theoretically, humoral therapy was tailored to the habits and disposition of the patient and the extent of the disease. Therefore, the *hospitalière* had to be familiar with her patients and their various symptoms in order to make adequate reports to the surgeon and to tailor the treatment accordingly. Unfortunately, Bertin stated that most slaves experienced a reoccurrence of the disease and many suffered the ill effects of crab yaws.

Some *hospitalières* ignored European remedies, and, instead, offered therapies formulated by slaves. One preparation to treat yaws involved combining sarsaparilla, unrefined sugar, and water and allowing it to steep and ferment. The patient then consumed the preparation and limited himself to dry foods like biscuits. According to Ducoeurjoly, the remedy resulted in a complete cure in forty days. In addition to the limited dietary regimen, the patient was to be bathed. The slave therapy appealed to both the slaves and their masters. Enslaved men and women were likely familiar with it, while their masters were no doubt pleased to learn that the slaves continued to work instead of being confined to the yaws hut during the course of the treatment.[48]

The *hospitalière* also cared for the *nouveaux* (new slaves). She was responsible for providing new slaves with appropriate care and extra food in order to ensure that they survived the crucial first year.[49] The new slaves were fed *à la main*; in other words, the planter provided the slaves with cooked food. Some plantations had rooms set aside for storing the vegetables and other essentials. In this way, new slaves were not forced to grow and cook their own food immediately. The *nouveaux* eventually learned how to cultivate crops produced on the plantation on a piece of ground set aside for that purpose. After about eight months of this instruction, under the guidance of another slave, the new slave would be absorbed into the general population and be responsible for *grand travaux*, or field labor.[50]

LeCesne's correspondence with his employers revealed his efforts to ensure the survival of newly arrived slaves. In September 1790 LeCesne wrote that the fourteen slaves (seven men and seven women) he had bought for his employers' plantation were in excellent physical health. In order to allay the concerns of his bosses and justify the purchases he made, he reassured them that "The slaves are fine, vigorous, robust, and healthy; the first choice of a cargo that did not have a single sick slave." He expressed his hope that before a year had passed they would be acclimated and ready to work with the other slaves. LeCesne never failed to mention these slaves in the correspondence that followed and the progress they were making. He did admit, however, that, like all *nouveaux*, they were "paying their dues to the climate but were nevertheless managing to endure."[51]

In addition to preparing and distributing food to the *nouveaux*, the *hospitalière* participated in inoculation procedures to prevent smallpox outbreaks. Smallpox was a great killer in Saint Domingue, and the constant influx of people to the island brought fresh contagion as well as victims.[52] In 1772, for example, an epidemic, believed to have begun as a result of infection aboard a slave ship, killed more than 1,200 people in Cap-François.[53]

In order to combat the disease, some residents practiced inoculation. After 1768 R.-N. Joubert de la Motte, a physician, royal botanist, and director of the royal botanical gardens in Port-au-Prince, vigorously promoted the technique. His high standing within the medical and scientific community of Saint Domingue gave greater credibility to a procedure that continued to have many critics during the course of the eighteenth century. The Paris medical faculty endorsed inoculation only in the 1760s, nearly twenty years after the procedure was first attempted in Saint Domingue. The exceptional references to the uses of the method by physician J.-L. Polony on himself, his wife, and his family in 1771 and by other whites point to the limited practice of inoculation among European and white Creole residents of Saint Domingue.[54]

In 1774 Arthaud continued the fight to employ inoculation as a way to prevent the suffering and death that resulted from smallpox epidemics in the colony. He wrote a pamphlet to encourage colonists to have themselves, their children, and their slaves inoculated. Arthaud pointed out that theologians were the most vociferous critics of the procedure, and he disputed their claim that the technique was a form of homicide. He said that the clergy's position was fatalistic and endangered the practice of medicine. He indicated that "The Chinese, whose political administration has astonished us and whose wisdom and knowledge we have admired, have used it for more than a century. The English, who live in a country where right sense dominates, practice it."[55] Arthaud's implication was subtle yet clear: France was being held back by the superstitious beliefs of its religious leaders while the most powerful and revered nations in the world utilized the technique.

The most positive publicity that the medical technique received resulted from the efforts of Simeon Warlock, a Creole resident of Antigua and brother-in-law of Daniel Sutton, the English inoculator. After arriving in Saint Domingue in 1774, Warlock proceeded to inoculate thousands of slaves in the area of Quartier-Morin. The procedure's low cost, combined with Warlock's reputation as a man of high character, went a long way in convincing planters and their managers to practice the method on their plantations.[56]

Sources show that managers confined the slaves who were to receive inoculation at the plantation hospital or in the yaws hut. Young Creole slaves, as well as the *nouveaux*, were generally chosen for the procedure because they likely had not experienced the disease and, therefore, had no immunity to it. In addition, the *nouveaux* and the young represented an increase in the slave population, and planters had invested much money in order to see the ranks of their workforce increased.[57] They did not want their investment depleted by smallpox. Countess d'Agoult's plantation hospital journal from May 1789 shows the admission of fifteen slaves to the hospital for inoculation. Only one out of the fifteen slaves was an adult, an Ibo man who served as a *sucrier* (a valuable worker involved in the production and processing of sugar cane). Countess Agoult's manager, Genton, may have decided to inoculate the slaves after hearing word of smallpox outbreaks on neighboring plantations.[58] Such news convinced many managers to inoculate slaves who had not contracted the disease. Plantation manager Planteaux, like LeCesne, managed a plantation for the Counts Vaudreuil and Duras. His efforts to prevent the outbreak of smallpox proved futile in May 1789. After inoculating both male and female slaves, Planteaux learned that two new slaves, a man and woman, had already contracted the disease. According to Planteaux's letters from July and August, the appearance of the disease on the plantation at Morne Rouge in northern Saint Domingue resulted in the admission of many slaves to the plantation hospital and eventually the deaths of two female slaves from the disease. Attempting to put a positive spin on the loss of two workers, Planteaux wrote that he "was happy not to have lost more because there were plantations that had lost up to fifteen slaves."[59] LeCesne, who no doubt had learned of Planteaux's failure, reassured his employers in a letter dated 11 May 1790 that he would be inoculating about thirty slaves if the smallpox that gripped neighboring plantations was to appear at the plantation in Cul-de-Sac.[60]

Inoculation and slavery advanced simultaneously because inoculation provided a low-cost method of ensuring the survival of one's slave, while slavery furnished the bodies required for the development and refinement of the inoculation technique. Physicians and surgeons had a large captive population on which to practice what was by European standards a controversial medical procedure. Physicians had no qualms about practicing an experimental medical procedure like inoculation on African and Creole slaves because, according to medical notions of the day, blacks experienced little or no pain. Moreau de Saint-Méry noted that "the slave women give birth with great ease."[61] Physicians, likewise, reminded planters that the biological makeup of the African and Afro-Caribbean suited them for hard labor under a hot sun.[62] According to these Western medical practitioners, the slight incision necessary to inoculate the slave would be painless.

One should not look at inoculation, however, as the advancement of medical science only at the expense of the slave and the invasion of his or her body. Inoculation may have commanded more widespread and earlier acceptance in Saint Domingue because the population on which the

method was employed was already familiar with the technique and practiced it among themselves.[63] Inoculation in Saint Domingue represents
the influence and appropriation of African medical techniques into the
Western medical canon. Eighteenth-century German naturalist Paul Erdman Isert wrote that although smallpox existed among an African people known as the Akreens or Gah it was not murderous because they
practiced inoculation. He reported, "During my whole trip, I saw no one
develop the disease naturally, and am persuaded that because inoculation is as ordinary here as circumcision this disease will end entirely."[64]

A story related by Charles Arthaud demonstrates that inoculation,
a form of indigenous medical knowledge, survived the Middle Passage
and came to be used by African slaves not only among themselves and
on their children but also on the children of their masters. Arthaud wrote:
"A *Dame* assured me of having been inoculated in her youth along with
seven slave children by a male slave who had practiced this method in
Africa. The slave made a superficial incision on the inner thigh with a
razor and put in the incision some varolic pus. The *Dame* . . . told me
that she had a very benign case of smallpox as did the children with
whom she had been inoculated."[65] Arthaud's inclusion of this story
should not be viewed as praise for the accomplishments of African men
and women. In the same pamphlet in which he extolled Chinese and English men and women for their practice of inoculation, he remarked that
Africans, likewise, performed the technique. He argued that if such a simple people used the therapy, then the French should do the same.

Slaves called their inoculation procedure *acheter la petite vérole*
(buying smallpox). Physician Duchemin de l'Étang explained that the
slaves referred to inoculation in this way "because those from whom
they get it sell it to them who want to give it to themselves." De l'Étang
meant that certain slaves were involved in the sale, or, at least, the distribution of smallpox pus and scabs.[66] The buying and selling of smallpox was customary for the residents of northeastern Africa. On learning
that smallpox existed in the area, women traveled to the location and
sought out victims of the disease. Finding an infected child, the woman
proceeded to wrap cloth around the arm of the diseased, bargained with
the child's mother over the price of the pocks, and then returned home
in order to tie the cloth around her own child.[67]

The Infirmière

Infirmières assisted the *hospitalière*. These young women normally prepared baths, washed the linen of the patients, and cared for the babies

whose mothers worked in the fields and for orphan children. The *infirm-ière* also served as the *commandeuse*, or the female driver of the third field gang. Children between the ages of eight and thirteen were the members of this work gang, who were responsible for picking weeds and gathering cane trash. Planters selected women on the basis of their ability to care for and discipline children and for their medical talents. In particular, the women had to be able to effectively treat chigger infestation and infection, detect and prevent pica, and bathe the children.[68] Unlike the *hospitalière*, the aide was not considered among the highest-ranking slaves but instead held the status of an *ouvrière*, or worker. Despite the lower status, the *infirmière* was often singled out for her efforts. Lory de la Bernardière, an absentee proprietor from Nantes, noted in correspondence to his son that he was happy to hear that the hospital aide, Julie, had provided life-saving care to slaves attacked by smallpox during the epidemic of 1774.[69]

The Midwife

A slave midwife also worked on the plantation. Like the *hospitalière*, the midwife was an important member of the slave hierarchy. The midwife's main responsibilities were to assist slave women in labor and to provide postnatal care to the mother and child. Slave midwives knew how to treat gynecological and obstetric ailments by means of herbal remedies.[70]

The role of the midwife became very important during the Seven Years' War (1756–63), a conflict that wreaked havoc on the colonial economy. The imperial contest pitted France against Britain, combatants that fought over territory on the American mainland, in the Caribbean, and Asia. Britain, the dominant power on the high seas, prevented French shippers from reaching the island with much-needed goods, including slaves from Africa. To make matters worse, the British captured Senegal and Gorée, the largest of France's slave-trading areas. The smugglers, likewise, found it difficult to supply the colony. As a result of the trade blockade and the unavailability of cheap food sources, slaves starved and agricultural production fell.[71] The arrival of slaves from the coasts of Africa was no longer sufficient and the price of new slaves increased dramatically. As a result, planters were forced to depend on natural increase, a significant change in plantation administration. Before 1760 colonists saw reproduction as a serious economic drain because pregnancy diminished the amount of work that could be completed by enslaved women. In addition, proprietors resented the children produced because, in the minds of the planters, they did little work and were nothing more than extra mouths to feed.[72] After 1760 slavery advocates concerned themselves with reproduction because they viewed female slaves as breeding units that were not living up to their full reproductive potential. Writing in the 1780s, proprietor Stanislas Foäche maintained, "Births must replace deaths. The small number of children born to the slaves is always surprising. . . . [G]ood administration . . . will be able to increase the population." Appealing to the economic interest of his fellow planters, Foäche claimed that Creole slaves were more productive than those from Africa: "Not only are the Creole slaves better than those from Guinea, but they also form families that are rooted to the land and, therefore, easier to control. There is no comparison between the work of the old work gangs [composed of African slaves] and that completed by new slaves." Foäche felt the need to convince other proprietors of the wisdom of natural increase because he realized that some of them still maintained the pre-1760s attitude that enslaved infants and children were economic burdens. He wrote, "They pretend that a Creole slave costs them too much in food and clothing, which they are obliged to furnish before the slave will be able to work, and by the loss of the mother's work when she nurses. They are deceiving themselves greatly."[73] Without a constant supply of slave bodies, the social and economic systems of the colony were in jeopardy.

Some plantation managers practiced positive reinforcement in order to raise birth rates among slaves. They rewarded midwives, as well as new mothers, with small gifts at the birth of a healthy newborn and then again when the child celebrated its third month of life. Money and fabric were the most common inducements given to midwives and mothers. Some plantation managers exempted midwives from hard labor and mothers received days off from work in proportion to the number of children they gave birth to. Still other midwives and fruitful mothers received *la liberté de la savane*, a type of limited unofficial freedom by which the planters avoided paying an administrative *taxe d'affranchissement* (manumission tax) to the government. Slaves who had been granted *la liberté de la savane* continued to live on the plantation, received rations from the master, and tended their own gardens but had the freedom to come and go as they pleased, to work if they wanted, and to participate in the social life of the plantation. These slaves became known as *libres de fait*. They normally cultivated larger garden plots, sold the excess produce, and achieved a level of economic freedom, which may have ultimately translated into *libre de droit,* or complete freedom, for themselves or a relative. Planters also rewarded the children of domestic slaves like midwives with *libre de fait* by sending the children to France or to another colony to learn a trade.[74] Medical skills, such as midwifery, were usually passed

from a female to a younger female relative. Planters concerned with na-
tality rates on their plantations may have sent the young relative of a
skilled midwife to one of Saint Domingue's urban areas to hone the skills
she had learned from the older, more experienced relative. *Hospitalières*
also had the opportunity to achieve the status of *libre de fait;* the fact that
Mary Louise Vermandois, one of the three *hospitalières* on the Duras and
Vaudreuil plantation, was listed with a last name may be evidence that
she was a *libre de fait.*

Although midwives were prized members of the slave hierarchy, they
were at the same time viewed with great suspicion. Planters and white
medical practitioners accused midwives of murdering newborn infants in
order to free them from a life of slavery. They also were charged with destroying fetuses by means of herbal abortifacients.[75] Pouppée-Desportes
presented evidence that shows that slave women possessed information
about plants capable of inducing abortions. Pouppée-Desportes's work on
medical botany included a recipe for a tea that promised to reestablish
menstruation. By restoring menstruation, it also worked to terminate pregnancy. The main ingredients of this infusion were the leaves of the *avo-
catier (laurus persea)*, or the avocado tree. Pouppée-Desportes mentioned
that this tree and its leaves were "the universal remedy of the slaves for
female complaints."[76] In Cuba today, traditional healers boil the leaves of
the purple varieties of this tree, or three new shoots of any variety, to form
a decoction that is consumed in order to bring on an abortion.[77]

Proprietors also believed that midwives were responsible for spreading *mal de mâchoire* or *tétanos*, a condition that was most likely tetanus
when the term was applied to adults and either neonatal tetany or
tetanus when applied to children. Dazille claimed that midwives used
mysterious means, which they refused to reveal even under threat of torture. Medical practitioners also argued that the umbilical cord was the
most common site of infection because of the rusty instruments used to
cut the cord.[78] Some supposed that midwives spread the disease unin-
tentionally by using a burnt rag to tie the cord and not examining it for
nine days, a practice derived from African custom and reportedly still
employed in Haiti today.[79]

As a result of these negative views, some planters punished midwives
whom they perceived as malicious by whipping both them and the mothers when infants died, or by forcing them to wear an iron collar until the
mothers became pregnant again.[80] A midwife named Arada who lived on
the Fleuriau plantation wore a rope collar with seventy knots, the number of children she was believed to have killed. A lawyer representing
Madame Dumoranay, owner of two plantations, advised the proprietor to

get rid of one of her midwives, an enslaved woman blamed for many deaths.[81] Other planters and their employees restricted the role played by the female slave attendant in the birthing process. A male medical practitioner, usually the plantation surgeon, began to replace the midwife or at least usurp her authority at the bedside during the closing decades of the eighteenth century. The power of French and white Creole midwives in Saint Domingue, as well as that of their counterparts in Europe, had already deteriorated by this time. Armed with new methods and tools (like the forceps), surgeons and physicians now assumed control of labor and delivery. These changes tended to be based on class; women of higher economic standing were the first to have the births of their children supervised by male surgeons or male midwives.[82] This explains why slaves were among the last to experience transformations in the role of the midwife. Dazille supported the exclusion of women (whether white or black, free or slave) from the bedchamber and recommended that the royal physician of the colony teach surgical students the proper way to care for women in all stages of pregnancy. Dazille also recommended that proprietors require surgeons to visit pregnant women every eight days. Dazille devoted an entire work to the study of pregnancy.[83]

It was economically undesirable, however, to call for a plantation surgeon every time a slave delivered a child. Instead of eliminating the midwife, some physicians, like Jean-Damien Chevalier, recommended that "a capable Surgeon show the slave midwives the manner of tying off the umbilical cord."[84] Chevalier's suggestion is revealing not only of European medical attitudes toward untrained midwives but also testifies to the lack of confidence that physicians had in many plantation surgeons. Chevalier does not simply say that a surgeon is necessary but that a capable one must be the instructor.

Just as the sick were housed in the plantation hospital and those suffering from yaws resided in the yaws hut, pregnant slaves were taken to a special lying-in hospital. Planters and their employees hoped that this building would prevent women from being exposed to unhealthy air. They also recommended that newborns be held in these hospitals for at least nine days in order to avoid contracting *tétanos*.[85]

The Plantation Healers: Accommodation and Resistance

Of all the enslaved healers, plantation women seemed to be those healers who accommodated the desires and goals of the white managers and his planter employers. Enslaved female medical workers healed the sick who would again work for the master and adhered to the idea of the plantation hospital as a place of correction. This accommodation, of course, was co-erced, often through physical punishment. At the same time, the *hospi-talières, infirmières,* and midwives actively undermined and resisted slav-ery by retaining African medical traditions, fashioning an Afro-Caribbean health system, assuming leadership roles in their community, allowing those pretending to be ill to remain within the plantation hospital to avoid work, providing infant care to expectant mothers, supplying the same women with abortions, and participating in acts of infanticide.[86]

By caring for the ill, *hospitalières, infirmières,* and midwives sup-ported the slave system. Their recommendations and reports made to the plantation surgeon determined who was fit to labor in the fields or at other more skilled tasks. They also helped the planters to retain money that would be lost in buying slaves to replace those who had died from disease. One sees evidence for this last fact most clearly in inoculation procedures in which *hospitalières* took part. Similarly, the skillful work of midwives provided planters with newborn laborers.

Female medical workers also put into practice the planter's ideology of care. They were ordered to make visits to the plantation hospital as quick and as unappealing as possible by using restraints and by follow-ing closely the regimen prescribed by the plantation surgeon. Similarly, midwives on some plantations followed the overseers' commands to re-port pregnancies and enclose women in lying-in hospitals where they would be subject to the demands of a surgeon-midwife, not surrounded by female friends and relatives.

Conversely, *hospitalières, infirmières,* and midwives emerged as sig-nificant leaders of slave communities through a process of cultural reten-tion, assimilation, and creation. Their labor allowed them to retain ele-ments of African healing traditions and to contribute to the creation of an Afro-Caribbean health care system.[87] Women's employment as enslaved healers echoed African social roles. Within African medical structures, women enjoyed status as healers; in Sierra Leone, for example, women's participation in healing was greatly respected.[88] Their positions made them leaders of the slave community, especially among slave populations that were overwhelmingly African and not Creole.

The enslaved healers also participated in occupational sabotage; in other words, they used their positions to interfere with the productivity of the plantation and the work completed there. *Hospitalières* took part in occupational sabotage by allowing malingerers to remain within the walls of the plantation hospital long after their "illnesses" had been cured. After caring for the sick for many years, *hospitalières* easily differentiated between the truly ill and those feigning illness. Their complicity in these acts of deception compounded the negative consequences for the master. The slave was not working, needed rest was made available to the malingerer, and extra food and medicines were expended. The high rank that the *hospitalière* held meant that she could demand food and supplies from the planter's storehouse.[89] Moreover, the psychological satisfaction that both "patient" and *hospitalière* received from deceiving the master or his employee was, no doubt, exhilarating. An excellent example of a *hospitalière's* involvement in a case of feigned illness is the story of a slave woman named Francine who, in the words of the plantation overseer Dujardin de Beaumetz, "had been in the convalescence house for centuries for an incurable ulcer."[90] An unnamed *hospitalière* surely administered and permitted Francine's admittance and lengthy stay in the plantation hospital. Like female medical workers in other French colonies, *hospitalières* in Saint Domingue had ready access to medicines and herbs that they used as poisons. In Martinique, *hospitalière* Magdeleine used drugs as poisons in order to keep control over other domestic servants, to influence who was named to key posts in the slave hierarchy, and to terrorize the whites who managed the plantation on which she worked.[91]

Finally, *infirmières* and midwives had ample opportunity to engage in occupational sabotage. Midwives possessed knowledge about plants that could be used to bring on an abortion and employed them. They assisted mothers in acts of infanticide. Through their work as *commandeuses*, *infirmières* had control over the labor of the third field gang and could limit the productivity of this group as needed.

4 Enslaved Herbalists

> The slaves know how to make the most of all the plants
> that Nature has strewn freely in this rich climate. It is
> fortunate when they only make use of them to provide re-
> lief from infirmities! But, unfortunately, they sometimes
> abuse them.
>
> —Nicolas Bourgeois, *Voyages Intéressans*, 1788

On the plantations and in the marketplaces of Saint Domingue, slaves and even white colonists found enslaved men and women renowned for their abilities to cure ailments by means of herbal remedies. These herbalists treated dreadful wounds, raging fevers, and frightening cases of scurvy with plants they gathered along the riverbanks and in the wilds. They drew upon traditional African herbalism, information gleaned from native Caribbeans, and their own practical experience to offer aid to their fellow bondsmen and to European and white Creole residents. Motivated by their desire to uncover the next big medical cure, French physicians and scientists eagerly sought out these men and women. They hoped to learn about and convey to their readers in both word and image the herbal therapies employed by enslaved men and women and native Caribbeans. But, as the quote from Bourgeois shows, the whites of Saint Domingue also eyed the herbalists nervously because along with their ability to heal came the potential to harm.

Conquering and Colonizing Saint Domingue's Plant Kingdom

The Western project to locate and employ remedies from foreign pharmacopoeias occupied an important place in the colonizing projects of European nations. In speaking about the Torrid Zone, Ducoeurjoly reported, "The three kingdoms of nature, animal, vegetable and mineral, there offer the most marvelous specifics."[1] The Europeans who conquered the New World were not only interested in subduing native peoples and exploiting African slaves but also were engaged in discovering, understanding, and profiting from new plant and animal sources. The search for medical miracles followed the mercantilist philosophy that motivated European nations. The knowledge possessed by herbalists and the plants they employed in their recipes functioned as natural resources for European researchers, who through a process of scientific production sought to transform the resources into refined commodities. Thus, French colonists not only exploited the manual labor of African and Afro-Caribbean slaves, but also mined their cultural systems for medical treasures from which the French profited. Yet like the machetes that slaves used for both labor and as weapons against other slaves and white slaveholders, herbal remedies sometimes were transformed from means of curing to ways of killing.

The search for new therapies figured prominently in the iconography that accompanied the efforts to establish colonies in the New World. For centuries, many scholars compared the New World to Christianity's Garden of Eden and hoped that the plants, animals, and minerals found there could be used to cure disease. According to colonial ideology and iconography, slaves and native Caribbeans offered Europe their medicinal and natural treasures; Europe, on the other hand, presented them with finished products as well as refined intellectual works. Visual allegories supported the mercantilist policies of European nations, symbolized the imperialistic scientific and medical research undertaken by European scholars, and represented Europe's vision of the political positions of the various actors in the New World drama.

An excellent French example of this colonial vision is the frontispiece of Jean-Baptiste Dutertre's *Histoire Général des Antilles* (Figure 5). In this work, one sees Nature joining France and the New World and pointing to the goods that each people will provide to the other. France, represented as a man of the upper class, receives the natural treasures of the Caribbean—plants, woods, and exotic creatures like the tortoise and the armadillo. These items pour forth from a cornucopia. The peoples of the Caribbean, represented as both a man and a woman, accept finished products—combs, scissors, weapons, tools, barrels, and bales of materials. It is interesting that the artist added a book; while the Caribbean people provided scientific raw material, Frenchmen supplied the finished scientific product. Dutertre's allegorical frontispiece is an excellent summary

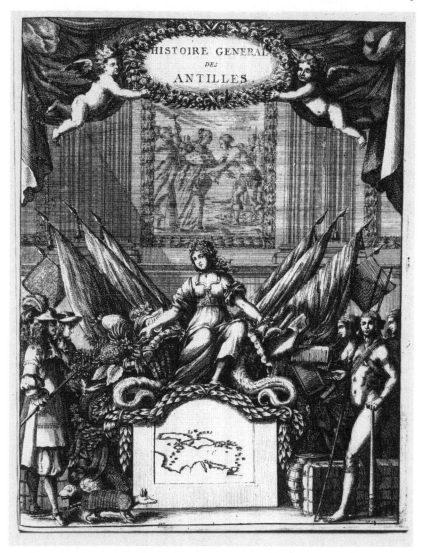

Figure 5. Frontispiece to Jean-Baptiste Dutertre's Histoire Général des Antilles *(Paris, 1667). Courtesy the Newberry Library, Chicago.*

of his text, which consists of essays describing New World plants, animals, and the herbal cures employed by the natives of the Antilles.

Iconographic frontispieces employed gendered and racial symbols to indicate the power relationships that existed between the Old and New Worlds, their inhabitants, and the resources each offered. The engraver chose to represent the New World as both male and female and the Old World as male for a number of reasons. One explanation is the important role that native Caribbean women reportedly played in the gathering, preparation, and distribution of healing plants. In fact, Dutertre asserted, "The women have greater knowledge of the qualities of plants . . . than the men, and they make use of this knowledge."[2] Dutertre's assessment of the contribution of Caribbean women to the native pharmacopoeia also likely was influenced by European herbal tradition. European female healers possessed great knowledge of the curative powers of herbs. They employed them in their work as midwives, herbalists, and cooks. Men and women consulted women across the socioeconomic spectrum for herbal advice. They depended on the village gentlewoman as well as the old widow who lived on the outskirts of town to offer relief.[3]

Another explanation for the difference in the gendering of the figures is that the colonization projects of the European nations were overwhelmingly male. For much of the history of Saint Domingue, the population of European and white Creole women remained small in comparison to the number of white men. The engraver's decision to portray European colonists as male also related to a trend in European science to describe the discovery and development of scientific theories and products in terms of birth and reproduction. Unlike the production of human creatures, the progeny created by the new science resulted only from the male seed. In other words, men of science and learning described their production of texts, ideas, theories, and items as a type of birth in which they solely took part. They looked to and expanded upon older notions of masculine creation, including Aristotelian reproduction, Judeo-Christian legends, and alchemical writings. All three traditions emphasized the ability of the male or masculine force to work with feminine nature and to produce without a female partner. Aristotle affirmed that the male contribution to reproduction was more substantial than the female. According to him, the male provided the form, or what was necessary for development and generation, while the female simply supplied the matter on which to build and act. The Jewish and Christian faiths both credited the formation of the universe to a male deity. The descent of the Holy Spirit embodied in a pure white dove overshadowed the Virgin's role as a simple receptacle or vessel.[4] Likewise, alchemists emphasized the primacy of the male contribution to creation—Sole (the sun) or the masculine creative principle overshadowed the female creative force, Luna (the moon). Alchemists not only stressed the masculine role in alchemical metaphysics, but their greatest proponent, Paracelsus, believed that humanlike beings could be formed without the involvement of a female organism.[5]

Race also was a significant element in Dutertre's frontispiece. The picture clearly divides the peoples of the Old World from those of the New. In addition, the painting that hangs above Nature displays the submissive attitude expected of Native Caribbeans by Europeans. The representative of the native peoples bows respectfully in front of European political and religious authorities. Finally, the enslaved man who looks out from behind the European gentlemen presages the important part that enslaved men and women played in the transfer of knowledge between the Old World (Europe and Africa included) and the New World. His supporting role in the illustration indicates the position of slaves in the imperialistic efforts of Europe—foundational but intentionally forgotten.

Who Were the Enslaved Herbalists?

Enslaved herbalists were respected members of the slave community. Both men and women served as enslaved herbalists; many likely combined their herbal expertise with other types of medical care. As we have seen, *hospitalières* and midwives utilized herbal remedies; healers who specialized in spiritual medicine, like divination and the selling of charms and spells, also employed herbalism. Documents do record instances when a specific man or woman is consulted because of his or her skill in treating a particular ailment. Often, however, Europeans simply said that slaves knew how to treat this condition or that disease; they did not tend to differentiate one enslaved person from another—they did not see them as individuals. Some of the remedies might, however, have been so common that many slaves were aware of them and freely used them.

The enslaved herbalists to whom French researchers referred were also expected characters in an Enlightenment story. Over the course of the eighteenth century, physicians and scientists spoke of nameless men and women who possessed nature's secrets. Often these remedies were diffused via a well-placed European woman, like Lady Mary Wortley Montagu and the Ana de Osorio, countess of Chinchón. These mysteries were then subjected to the trials imposed and expected by the new science. The stories of the great remedies usually included the intrepid and curious scientist and the native healer, village woman, or, in the case of Saint Domingue, enslaved herbalist. Consider the native healer who shared the secret of cinchona with the early explorers of the New World, the old neighborhood woman from whom William Withering received the herbal concoction from which digitalis was extracted, and the milkmaids who conveyed to Edward Jenner the knowledge that a bout of cowpox protected one from the ravages of smallpox.[6] Were these untrained

yet experienced individuals real people? Are these stories historically accurate and verifiable? Yes, but the accounts are also testaments to an
age's search for truth about and by way of the natural world. The Enlightenment saw simple men and women of a lower class or members of
different races as closer to nature and even part of nature itself.

By including nature's messengers like the enslaved herbalists in their
discovery narratives, the physicians of Saint Domingue and scientists elsewhere were not only responding to and incorporating Enlightenment imagery but also drew their inspiration from a less intellectual, less honor-
able arena. They took as their example the remedy peddlers who hawked
cure-alls atop wagons in small European villages and crowded cities.
These mountebanks often spoke of exotic persons from whom they received their special tonics.[7] Not only did the learned and degreed physicians in the colony utilize the charlatan's old marketing trick, but colonial drug sellers took advantage of it as well. One remedy retailer revealed
to his potential customers that his cure for venereal ailments came from
a native inhabitant of the Gold Coast of Africa who exchanged the recipe
for the druggist's gold and a vow to keep secret the remedy until the
Frenchman left the shores of Africa.[8]

Just as the colonial drug seller looked to Africa for inspiration, enslaved herbalists drew upon their African origins to heal with herbs.
Slaves born in Africa made up the largest portion of the Saint Domingue
population; therefore, the herbalism being formulated by slaves in Saint
Domingue was constantly being renewed and reinforced with ideas and
information brought by the *nouveaux*. African healing traditions were
very old, reaching back thousands of years before the Common Era. Ancient African kingdoms and empires possessed elaborate healing systems,
the most famous being that articulated and documented by the Egyptians.
Healers utilized diverse natural objects, including plants, minerals, and
animals, in their healing procedures. Believing that illness resulted from
either natural or divine causes, African herbalists treated these sicknesses
with herbal remedies and by practicing divination.[9] Practitioners not only
recognized that plants, animals, and minerals were essential components
in healing remedies, but also emphasized that these items were important cultural symbols. A plant's ritual significance could not be separated
from its healing ability. African men and women also did not differentiate between plants as drugs and plants as food sources—plants were consumed for their health benefits.[10] Europeans who reported on the healing
activities of slaves did note that food was an essential part of the slaves'
medical system but did not mention and likely did not understand the
symbolic qualities of the herbs.

African slaves also incorporated elements of native Caribbean herbalism into their healing repertoire. Recall that Dutertre said that native women knew more about herbs and their medicinal uses than male Caribbeans; he mentioned that women employed herbs to treat infertility and to ease the pains of childbirth.[11] Men known as *butio*s also were responsible for the practice of medicine, surgery, and pharmacy among the native Caribbeans. The medical aid they furnished normally encompassed both supernatural intervention and herbal therapy. *Butio*s would seek the assistance of Caribbean gods called *Zémè*s on behalf of the ill. The response of the *Zémè*s would then be interpreted dramatically by the *butio*. If he appeared joyful and danced, the answer was positive, but if he was sad, then the request had been denied.[12]

Like Dutertre, European medical scholars and practitioners of the eighteenth century continued to look to native Caribbeans, to documents about their history, and to enslaved herbalists for indigenous remedies that might be used to treat diseases both in the colony and in Europe. Pouppée-Desportes wrote, "The first Europeans who lived in America, having been afflicted with sicknesses that were unknown to them, had recourse to the remedies of the natives of the country whom they called *Sauvages* (savages)."[13] Pouppée-Desportes reported that he scrutinized old texts for medical information but said that earlier colonial authors provided inexact and confusing botanical descriptions. Pouppée-Desportes was hopeful that his work might make plain the knowledge that the native Caribbeans possessed. In order to accomplish this goal, he included a catalog of plants, with Carib, French, and Latin names, in the third volume of his work on the diseases of Saint Domingue. Antoine Martinet, a Saint Domingue surgeon and pharmacist, also believed that the native *indiens* possessed great knowledge about herbs and medicinal plants; he even claimed that the Arawaks could distinguish beneficial plants from poisonous plants solely by sense of smell.[14]

One should not assume, however, that enslaved herbalists simply used plants from the African pharmacopoeia or merely imitated the remedies employed by native Caribbeans. The herbalism of the enslaved healers was undergoing dramatic changes in response to the new environment in which the slaves were thrust. They continued to make salves, lotions, and baths as their counterparts in Africa did, but the plants utilized were different. Herbal healers experimented with the plants that surrounded them. In fact, investigation into and experimentation with new plants were hallmarks of African herbalism. Some African herbalists did not train with an experienced teacher but instead relied upon dreams as sources of remedies.[15] They also relied upon an ancient theory known in Africa, Europe, and Asia. This theory, the Doctrine of the Signatures, taught that plants that resembled particular parts of the human body would effectively treat ailments associated with those body parts. In addition, the Yoruba people believed that possession by one of their deities caused a person to dart into the bush and collect plants, many of which might end up as part of the individual's personal supply of herbal remedies.[16]

The Search for the Next Big Cure

Much of what we know about the herbalists of Saint Domingue comes from French physicians who searched for herbal remedies employed by the African and Creole slave population. These men brought to life the visual allegories created by individuals like Dutertre. The slave herbalists sometimes revealed their remedies to prominent physicians, who then reported these recipes in medical books aimed at both European medical practitioners and the planter class. The most important of these French medical men were Nicolas Louis Bourgeois and Jean-Baptiste-René Pouppée-Desportes. Bourgeois served as secretary of the *Chambre d'Agriculture du Cap* in Saint Domingue, a royally sponsored agricultural society. His travel book about the Americas, *Voyages interessans dans différentes colonies françaises, espagnoles, anglaises,* contains a treatise on diseases common to Saint Domingue and the remedies employed to fight them. Bourgeois devoted a significant part of this memoir to his search for slave remedies and, like other eighteenth-century scholars in Saint Domingue, he convinced slave healers to reveal their therapeutic secrets to him. He noted that sometimes it was rather difficult to obtain information from the slave practitioners, perhaps because they feared retribution at the hands of legal authorities. He commented, "I have seen them practice other remedies, of which it was impossible to pull from them the secret. Perhaps someone will be more fortunate than I was. It is necessary to gain their confidence, as I was able to do with some of them, but their knowledge appears to follow no order and it derives from many countries; it is therefore hardly possible to systematize the knowledge that is scattered among them."[17] Pouppée-Desportes, likewise, searched for remedies among both the African and native Caribbean populations who inhabited Saint Domingue. The third volume of his multivolume work, *Histoire des Maladies de S. Domingue: Traité ou Abregé des Plantes Usuelles de S. Domingue,* provided descriptions of various plants and their uses.

According to the testimony of Bourgeois and Pouppée-Desportes, the herbalists treated a wide variety of physical ailments with herbal remedies. European researchers tended to record information that they hoped would be useful to three classes of readers: colonial slaveholders, white colonists in general, and men and women in France and other parts of Europe. They reported wound therapies to slaveholders who needed to deal with the accidental injuries and intentional physical harm that slaves experienced. Planters and their Creole and French workers were especially interested in dealing with *tétanos* and hoped that slave remedies might provide cures for this devastating disease. Authors like Bourgeois and Pouppée-Desportes also anticipated that the therapies might be employed in the treatment of the venereal disorders to which many colonists were subject. The mercury that Europeans used to treat venereal afflictions produced side effects that were often worse than the diseases. The plants that the slaves harvested might supply safer succor. Slaves also understood how to deal effectively with horrible febrile disorders like malaria and yellow fever that devastated European newcomers. Scurvy brought on by long voyages also laid waste to travelers, both white and black. Enslaved herbalists skillfully remedied the ravages that this condition created. Bourgeois hoped that his report of slave therapies might lead to drugs that could be transported easily to Europe and employed by sailors and others destined to travel on the high seas.

Wound Therapy

Enslaved herbalists recognized that some plants had qualities useful in wound care. This knowledge was practical because slaves faced the danger of injuring themselves every day. Sugar mill workers might have their hand or foot crushed by a roller, animal caretakers might be bitten or kicked by a mule or horse, and slaves daily risked cuts and bruises on their feet from going barefoot.[18] Hilliard d'Auberteuil reported that many slaves lost fingers "while putting sugar cane into the sugar mills."[19] Physical punishment, such as whippings, also resulted in dangerous, life-threatening wounds. Plantation overseers often employed a popular planter remedy, which called for a mixture of salt, cayenne, and lemon juice to be rubbed in the sores that lined the bodies of brutalized slaves. Dazille described this therapy: "When it happens that the manager or steward of a plantation is forced, for the sake of maintaining authority, to punish the slave by the whip . . . it is customary in some colonies to apply a mixture of lemon juice, sea salt, and red pepper on bloody wounds, immediately after punishment, to prevent suppurations, gangrene, and other unfortunate accidents."[20] Although this mixture may seem simply a form of torture, cayenne pepper is known to have pain-relieving qualities and may have aided healing.[21]

Motivated by the dangers they faced every day, the slaves employed their own system of wound care, which relied on an ointment made from *l'herbe-à-bled* (*Digitaria insularis:* sourgrass). Bourgeois noted that the slaves employed this herb in order to heal "contusions, bruises, abscesses, and wounds considered incurable by our pharmacy." He went on further to reveal that "they boil it . . . to form a sort of ointment that they apply to the wound, after having washed the wound with *tafia* [a type of alcohol consumed by the slaves]." They also used the leaf of the *langue-à-chat* (*Eupatorium odoratum*) to lessen the pain of bruises, contusions, and open sores. Scholars today conclude that *l'herbe-à-bled* and *langue-à-chat* have wound-healing abilities and report that they still are employed by the residents of the Caribbean for that purpose.[22]

Wound therapy also figured into the slaves' battle to avoid the dreaded disease tetanus. Such precautions sometimes proved inadequate and the slaves developed the disease. According to various accounts, the slave healers had a second line of medicinal defense against the disease and attempted to treat it by using various herbs. Well aware of the economic gain that a cure might bring, physicians and plantation surgeons searched for these therapies. Pouppée-Desportes wrote, "I wholeheartedly sought to discover the secret of a male slave who had a great reputation for treating [tetanus]."[23] Pouppée-Desportes noted that this herbalist tended to use liniments, infusions, poultices, and frictions as therapies. One popular liniment was made from *l'huile de palma Christi* (castor oil) (Figure 6). Physician Joseph Gardane reported, "In the method employed by the Blacks, against the spasm in general, or tetanus, one finds . . . liniment made with the grains of *palma Christi* (*Ricinus communis*), roasted, and pulverized." The white planters had taken to using the liniment as a form of preventive therapy in order to decrease the incidence of the affliction among newborn slaves. They "rub two or three times daily the temples and the jaws with the oil of *palma Christi.*"[24] The castor oil plant is of African origin. Thus, slaves applied African medical knowledge to the diseases they encountered daily in Saint Domingue.[25]

Slaves also learned some aspects of wound therapy from the indigenous peoples of the island (Figure 7). Pouppée-Desportes reported striking similarities between the remedies employed by slaves and those employed by native Caribbeans when treating puncture wounds of the foot. Both applied washes made of tobacco ashes to the sole of the foot in order to aid healing.[26] Bourgeois also mentioned that slaves employed tobacco and its juice quite effectively.[27] Historian Robert Voeks argues, "Even the medicinal use of some native American species, after being naturalized in Africa, diffused to the New World with the slave traffic. American to-

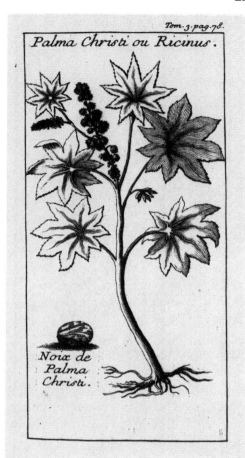

Figure 6. Palma Christi *(*Ricinus communis*), or the castor oil plant. Enslaved men and women used castor oil to treat tetanus.* Jean-Baptiste Labat, Nouveau Voyage aux Isles de l'Amérique *(The Hague, 1724), 3: 78. Used by permission of the Library Company of Philadelphia.*

bacco, for example, had arrived and was probably used medicinally in Africa by the 1600s."[28] Whether or not slaves possessed knowledge of medicinal tobacco prior to their arrival in the Caribbean or learned about its beneficial uses once there, it did make up an important part of their Afro-Caribbean medical arsenal. Besides utilizing tobacco as a form of wound therapy, native Caribbeans also employed *herbe des flèches* (herb of the arrow). Dutertre wrote, "The Savages have grand esteem for this plant, and not without reason, because we discovered . . . the rare and admirable qualities of which it is endowed: Its root, crushed and applied on wounds caused by arrows poisoned with Manchineel, kill the poison, stop gangrene from continuing, relieve inflammation."[29]

Enslaved herbalists did draw on their African medical knowledge and

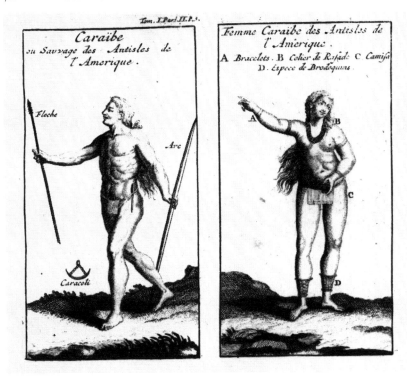

Figure 7. Caraïbe man and woman. Jean-Baptiste Labat, Nouveau Voyage aux Isles de l'Amérique *(The Hague, 1724), 1: 3. Used by permission of the Library Company of Philadelphia.*

on native Caribbean pharmacopoeia when dealing with wounds, bruises, and contusions, but they also innovated with plants found in Saint Domingue. They continued to make salves and lotions as their counterparts in Africa did, but the plants utilized were different. African folk practitioners made use of *Combretum glutinosum, Hibiscus asper,* and *Hyotis spicigera* when treating tetanus; these plants are not found in the Afro-Caribbean pharmacopoeia created by the enslaved herbalists.[30]

Fever Reducers

Enslaved herbalists also effectively treated fevers. French physicians were especially interested in finding new remedies for the various fevers that stalked the white residents of the island. The high incidence of malaria and yellow fever contributed to Saint Domingue's reputation as the Torrid Zone. Men like Bourgeois and Pouppée-Desportes sought out remedies that might be the next great pharmacological finding on a par with the discovery of cinchona, which had not only been a blessing to European colonization efforts by helping colonists survive their first days in the New World, but also proved a windfall to those who held a monopoly on the item.[31]

In a time when doctors called for bloodletting as a means of relieving the physical horrors inflicted by fever, the care provided by enslaved herbalists seems downright modern. Bourgeois reported that slaves generally treated fevers by bathing the sufferer in the coldest possible water and by applying cool, fresh herbs to the head. Slaves employed two types of herbs as febrifuges, *pourpier sauvage* and *herbe-à-piment.* The first was likely *Sesuvium portulacastrum,* more commonly known as purslane, a perennial herb that is still used in Haiti to treat fever by being either taken internally or applied externally.[32] Not satisfied with the reports of healing given him by the herbalists, Bourgeois confirmed the curative powers of these remedies by stating that he had seen trials conducted on whites that resulted in relief. The cold baths and herbal applications soon reduced their burning fevers and cleared their aching heads. Finally, like scientists before and after him, Bourgeois successfully tried the remedy on himself.[33]

Slaves also took herbal remedies internally in order to deal with fever. They made a decoction from *pois-puans* (literally, stinking peas; *Cassia occidentalis*). Bourgeois reported that the plant's name came from its foul stench. He indicated that slaves also roasted it and drank it as a type of coffee. It still is used for the same purposes in the Caribbean today.[34] Finally, Bourgeois noted that, although the slaves tended to use *pois-puans* as a febrifuge and as a basic component in their other medicinal infusions, he recommended it as a vermifuge as well.[35]

Antiscorbutic Remedies

Besides treating fevers and caring for wounds, enslaved herbalists also dedicated their practice to dealing with cases of scurvy. The poor and inadequate food provided by slave traders during the transport from Africa to the Caribbean meant that enslaved men and women suffered horribly from scurvy. In fact, it was one of the most common diseases among the *nouveaux.* Medical researchers like Bourgeois not only interested themselves in finding remedies utilized by slaves in order to share the information with slaveholding planters, but also to recommend therapies to the French navy and to travelers on the high seas.

One of the most important of the antiscorbutics advocated by the slaves was *cresson* (or cress). Enslaved herbalists applied various cresses in several ways. They advised their patients to rub the leaves in the mouth and to chew them in order to relieve abscesses in the mouth and throat. Slaves also incorporated the plant in their diets by adding it to salads and bouillons. Bourgeois noted that gums damaged and made rotten by scurvy and blemishes resulting from scurvy's effects readily responded to treatment with cress. He was so impressed by the efficacy of cress that he hoped that "a capable Chemist might extract a specific against scurvy from the plants . . . that could be transported beyond the seas."[36]

Taking Credit

Although eighteenth-century physicians, plantation surgeons, and white planters used slave remedies, they downplayed the role of the slave healer by placing the remedy within the traditional European therapeutic framework or by making reference to the healing traditions of esteemed nations. Gardane, for example, noted, "In Europe, following the doctrine of the father of medicine . . . they often have recourse to liniments . . . against spasmodic movements and pain caused by rheumatism."[37] Gardane discounted the herbalist's therapy against tetanus by noting that European practitioners who heeded the advice of Hippocrates utilized similar methods. Gardane referred to Hippocrates' prescription that stated, "When the case is such [tetanus follows a wound] treat the patient with vapour-baths, anoint him generously with oil, and warm him in firelight from a distance; anoint his body, and apply fomentation."[38] Similarly, Bourgeois sought to guarantee the efficacy of fever-reducing agents that slaves used by noting the successful cures experienced by whites, himself included. He also pointed out that medical men of the Orient recommended immersion in cool water. Arthaud used the same argument when making the case for inoculation in Saint Domingue. Bourgeois knew that his readers would place their trust in these techniques after learning that they were utilized by practitioners of one of the most ancient and respected medical systems in the world.[39]

Other physicians, for example, Dazille, simply rejected the remedies of enslaved herbalists. He was repulsed that respected medical practitioners sought out enslaved practitioners and used their herbal techniques. Dazille charged that Pouppée-Desportes had perpetrated a dangerous offense by offering the slave's remedy for tetanus. He argued that the colonial administrators had passed a "law by which it was prohibited to *gens de couleur* to treat tetanus, and to push their vulgar ignorance as far as torturing patients attacked by tetanus."[40] Dazille was referring to a 1764 law that prohibited "people of color or slaves from practicing medicine or surgery and treating any patients."[41] Dazille detested the practice of medicine by nonwhites. Dazille's criticism of Pouppée-Desportes appears ridiculous, however, when one considers that Pouppée-Desportes wrote the passage approximately sixteen years before the prohibition against black healers and practitioners of color was issued. Pouppée-Desportes's endorsement of the slave remedy, on the other hand, is characteristic of a life dedicated to the study of Saint Domingue's plants and the remedies that could be made from them.

To Harm as Well as to Heal: Herbalism as Political Resistance

In eighteenth-century Saint Domingue, physicians sought out enslaved herbalists in order to learn ways to deal with the devastating diseases that existed among both whites and blacks. But, as in other instances in the history of medicine, Western researchers took credit for the discovery of the information, and the contributions of enslaved men and women were obscured as their knowledge was subjected to the standards expected by the new science of the seventeenth and eighteenth centuries. As we will see in chapter 5 and by way of the story of one of the greatest enslaved healers, Makandal, the practice of herbalism by slaves was a powerful tool and a symbol of political resistance—that plants harmed as well as healed.

5 Makandal and the Medical Care of Animals: The Veterinarians Who Inspired the Haitian Revolution

> For over twenty-five years, the island of Saint Domingue shudders at the name of Makandal.
> —*Mercure de France,* 15 September 1787

In addition to providing care to human beings, enslaved healers also ministered to nonhuman creatures; in other words, some slaves practiced veterinary medicine.[1] Their work had significant economic, medical, social, and political consequences for slaves as well as for their European and Creole masters. Enslaved veterinary practitioners in eighteenth-century Saint Domingue contributed to the plantation economy and colonial prosperity, treated diseases that struck at both human and nonhuman populations, and ultimately inspired their fellow slaves to rebel against and overthrow French rule.

Animals in History

For centuries, humans, whether male or female, have been defined in relation to animals. Inspired by Plato, Greek philosophers affirmed humanity's transcendence of the natural world by devaluing the body. Taking their cue from Aristotle, other scholars sought to explain man's place within nature by reference to an organic model, which, nonetheless, acknowledged human superiority over nonhuman animals. The theory of the Great Chain of Being posited the existence of a ladder of nature on which various creatures, including man, were arrayed according to their level of perfection. Although man occupied the top of the ladder as a result of his *anima rationalis* (rationality), all creatures possessed *anima*, or the principle of life. Greco-Roman theorists, likewise, considered the differences between human and nonhuman animals. The most famous example of these considerations was Galen's *On the Usefulness of the Parts of the Body*, which argued that man's intelligence and ability to reason distinguished him from other creatures.[2] Medieval scholars remained enamored of classical philosophy; by combining it with Christian theology, they furthered the human and animal divide. Made in the image of the divine, man, who alone possessed a soul, had dominion over the other creatures. Unlike the medieval church authorities, practitioners of natural magic in the sixteenth and seventeenth centuries highlighted humanity's place within nature rather than above it, the presence of God in all creatures, and the dynamism of nature. With the onset of the Scientific Revolution in the seventeenth century, a mechanistic and materialistic worldview, which paid homage to the ideas of early Greek thinkers like Democritus, replaced the organic model. Man's superiority to the natural world was upheld by the unequal relationship between the scientific observer and natural objects, animals included. Cartesian mechanism furthered the devaluation of animals by arguing that they were nothing more than machines, devoid of feeling and, therefore, subject to experimentation and vivisection. Science became the pursuit of knowledge by the reasonable human, and animals became the objects of their studies. Inspired by René Descartes, scientific theorists denigrated the role of animals in nature, while practitioners of the anatomical sciences did the opposite. Comparative anatomy highlighted similarities in anatomical structure and led many scholars to question the sharp division of animal from man.[3]

Not only did early modern scientists weigh in on the human/nonhuman debate; political philosophers did likewise. Specifically, Thomas Hobbes depreciated the animal world as a dangerous and undesirable state. Without a strong sovereign, humans would be nothing but beasts. Humanity's existence would be "solitary, poor, nasty, brutish, and short"; in other words, it would be animal-like.[4]

The Enlightenment inherited the seventeenth century's increasing dissociation of human from nonhuman. The religious notion of the human's unique soul gave way to man's exceptional ability to reason. Man's rationality was not, like the eternal soul, a link to the divine; in fact, reason meant that man no longer needed even God.[5] The Scientific Revolution's legacy to the Enlightenment, however, was not accepted without dispute and controversy. Developments in the field of taxonomy questioned human exceptionality. The main advocate of the association of human with animal was Carolus Linnaeus, who placed the human creature on a par with the nonhuman animal in the first edition of *Systema Naturae* in 1735. Linnaeus boldly asserted that man was an animal, and that the science of natural history must include man as an object of investigation. As early as 1733, he had written in *Diaeta Naturalis*, "One should not vent one's wrath on animals. Theology decrees that a man has a soul and that the animals are mere *automata mechanica*, but I believe they would better advise that animals have a soul and that the difference is in nobility."[6] By linking man with animal, Linnaeus was not only showing the biological relationships between human and nonhuman creatures, but was also criticizing civilization. He wanted humanity to sincerely consider its place within nature and history and be open to the wisdom and moderation that animals exhibited. Enlightenment *philosophe* Jean-Jacques Rousseau also had much to say about humanity's connection to nature and the nonhuman creatures that inhabited it. Like Linnaeus, Rousseau urged his fellow human beings to identify with and look to animals for inspiration. He thought that the differences that existed between human and nonhuman animals had produced the despotism under which both now struggled. He asserted that the "voice of nature" was still present and could be heard via the human conscience.[7] An "Arcadian" view of nature exemplified by the life and written work of Englishman Gilbert White also characterized the relationship between humanity and the natural world in the eighteenth century. White sought and celebrated the connection between himself and his environment.[8] Materialists like Julien Offroy de La Mettrie, likewise, rejected the distinction between man and animal. La Mettrie wrote, "From animals to men, the transition is not violent." The materialists' repudiation of the break between humanity and the natural world harkened back to the ancient idea of the Great Chain of Being. Although creatures such as angels, humans, and animals were ranked, the divisions between them were blurred, and philosophers debated the distinction between instinct and reason. For some thinkers, not much difference existed; David Hume wrote, "Experimental reasoning [was] nothing but a species of instinct."[9]

As this brief survey shows, the association between humans and animals is not static and ahistorical. Some scholars rightly argue that it is affected by sociohistorical context as well as by constructions fashioned by humans. On the other hand, social constructionist approaches are, like any theories about human exceptionality, risky because they emphasize a unique quality that defines humanness—human ability to have culture and to give meaning and value to something through culture. Scholar Anna L. Peterson points out that "Most Western belief systems define humans as unique among the rest of life; humans are the only animal with x, an essential trait lacking in all other animals and setting people not only apart but also above them."[10] In order to avoid these dangers, my method of understanding the historical association between humans and animals can be defined as constrained constructionism, or, as articulated by Peterson, the view that "calls us to respect, take seriously, and seek out the viewpoints and the worlds shaped and inhabited not just by other humans but by a whole host of organisms sharing the planet. All these organisms are, like humans, embodied and embedded in the physical world. However, in various ways they are also all shapers of it, active agents and not merely blank paper waiting for human symbols and discourse . . . to make something of them."[11]

In addition to applying constrained constructionism to my study of the historical relationship between animals and humans in eighteenth-century Saint Domingue, I also am employing the notion of species as an analytical tool to get at the understanding of what it has meant to be human or animal across time. Just as race and gender have been used by historians and other scholars as instruments of critical inquiry, so too should the notion of species. By studying the relationship between human and nonhuman, we not only increase our knowledge of the past, but we also expand our understanding of race and gender, which have both been used to identify superior and inferior and influence the exercise of power. Peterson notes that the tendency to highlight how humans differ from nonhuman animals has been founded on the "logic of domination." In other words, differences are said to exist between human and nonhuman creatures, these differences become value laden, and they are then used to justify exploitation, not only of the environment but of other humans. As Peterson notes, "Many of these ideas about human nature are really about the particular kinds of humans who count, usually the same ones who have made the definitions."[12] The idea of women's inferiority, for instance, depended largely upon the fact that she was believed to be closer to nonhuman creatures. Women were unable to transcend their physicality, an activity that distinguished human from animal, because of the fact that they menstruated, gave birth, and lactated. For centuries, scholars had argued whether women possessed souls, and, therefore, whether they were fully human.

Animals and Saint Domingue

The significance of the interaction between animal and human subjects and its relationship to the development of France's most important colony cannot be overstated. Nonhuman animals played important roles in Saint Domingue's history—from its inception to the revolution that destroyed it. The colony's founding myth depended upon the legendary image of the adventuresome *boucanier* or the early settler who hunted and smoke-dried meats along the coasts of the Caribbean.[13] The tale of the *boucanier* appropriated two of the most masculine activities in Western culture—hunting and meat-eating—in order to highlight the power and authority of the early settler. One of the first chroniclers of life on the island of Saint Domingue, Alexander O. Exquemelin, wrote, "Each man flays the animals he has caught and removes the flesh from the bones. The meat is cut into strips about six feet long, sometimes more, sometimes less. The cut meat is strewn with ground salt and left in salt three or four hours. Then it is hung on sticks and beams. . . . They light a fire under it and smoke the meat."[14] The ability of the *boucanier* to hunt, kill, and consume meat affirmed his masculinity and power. In Exquemelin's description, "Immediately they have shot a beast, they take what they call their brandy—that is, they suck all the marrow from the bones before it is cold. . . . [B]ond-servants . . . prepare the food. This is always meat, for they eat nothing else."[15]

Since ancient times, hunting symbolized masculine power. Both Plato and Aristotle saw hunting as a way to exercise authority and highlight manly qualities. Both philosophers concentrated on the activity of hunting rather than its goal—the taking of a creature's life. For them, hunting was a process, a journey, and, ultimately, a means of self-identification. Aristotle taught that the power a hunter wielded over his prey was similar to the authority over "such of mankind designed for subjection." Since the medieval period, French monarchs and noblemen took to heart ancient teaching on the hunt. For them, the pursuit of prey was more than simple physical activity; instead, it was a performance designed to assert their power over the land, over animals, and most important, over their subjects.[16]

The *boucanier* was not only recognized for his skill as a hunter, but was also identified by his consumption of animal flesh. Like hunting, meat-eating has been a way to demonstrate one's superior place within society. Members of the upper classes had greater access to animal flesh, whether alive, in the midst of being hunted, or dead. The very definition of meat, "the essence or principal part of something," conveys authority and manliness. Meat's opposite, the lowly vegetable, was the food of choice for the poor and women. Its meaning, "suggesting passivity or dullness of existence, monotonous, inactive," likewise reinforces femininity and powerlessness. In times of want and war, meat is reserved for men, especially fighting men. Some scholars have pointed out that the act of hunting, an activity generally undertaken and completed by men, explains the relationship between power and meat consumption. Men, in other words, had control over an important economic commodity and its distribution.[17] The *boucanier*, the fabled hunter and meat-eater, became known as the founder of France's most productive slaveholding colony. The slaveholder embodied many of the qualities of the *boucanier*, specifically power over the life of a fellow creature.

Animals were not only central to the establishment of the colony but also essential to Saint Domingue's economic vitality. The value of a planter's estate not only included real estate, slaves, and luxury items, but also animals. According to Moreau de Saint-Méry, the animal population in northern Saint Domingue alone was "15,000 horses, 24,000 mules, and 88,000 other creatures including oxen, lambs, goats, and pigs."[18] Animals also fueled the economy because they played an integral part in transportation and the provision of power. Cattle pulled the carts that traveled across the plantations to the market towns and cities. Planters used animal power, specifically mules, in order to keep their milling operations moving. In fact, animal-driven mills outnumbered water mills 1,639 to 520.[19] Animal waste enriched the already productive soil of Saint Domingue. Laborie urged that "the dung of all kinds of cattle" and "the sweepings of pens, houses, kitchen, poultry, and pigeon houses" be collected and spread on the coffee fields.[20] Animal hides were among the major colonial export commodities. Nonhuman animals also provided food products; beef, sheep, goat, turkey, pigeon, and duck appeared on the colonial table.[21] In Saint Domingue, the preparation and distribution of meat were politically charged activities. The preparation of animal carcasses for meat production and leather fabrication devolved upon a social and racial class that was politically inferior to the whites: the *gens de couleur*, a group made up of free interracial men and women as well as free blacks. In 1776 the government stepped in and prohibited *gens de couleur* from selling meat believed to be tainted. Likewise, Spanish meat producers were accused of distributing spoiled and dangerous goods.[22]

In addition to playing a fundamental part in the market economy, animals figured into the scientific or intellectual economy of the French Empire. Naturalists established their scholarly reputations on the research they completed. Since the seventeenth century, natural historians concentrated on describing and analyzing the plant and animal life of the Caribbean. An excellent example is the Dominican priest, J.-B. Dutertre, who completed the four-volume *Histoire Générale des Antilles*. In both word and image, Dutertre set out to describe the diversity of animals and plants in the Antilles.[23] Over the course of the eighteenth century, European powers, France included, devoted much time, energy, and money to identifying plant and animal products that might turn out to be the next big colonial cash crop.[24]

What is most significant, animals provided the ideological rationale for the slave culture on which colonies like Saint Domingue were built. In other words, animals were used metaphorically to justify the enslavement of African men and women and their Creole descendants. From their initial capture, African men and women were treated as animals. Slave traders caught them and herded them toward the coasts, where they were confined until they were shipped to the colonies. Once they arrived, enslaved men and women were subjected to the prying eyes and hands of prospective owners, who tested their flesh to determine whether it was sound, strong, and healthy.[25] Within colonial literature, slaves were defined not as human creatures but as animals destined to work the fields. Labat wrote, "Slaves performed the work of horses, transporting merchandise from one place to the other." Girod-Chantrans also noted, "There is no domestic animal from which as much work is required as slaves and to which as little care is given."[26] The renaming of slaves with exotic or physically descriptive names furthered the animalization of enslaved men and women; the hot brand applied to the skin advanced the process of dehumanization. A striking example of the equation of slaves with animals can found as late as 1791 in the colonial newspaper *Affiches Américaines*. Advertisements announcing the sale of slaves, the majority of whom were branded, followed a notice about the escape of a mule with the brand "IN."[27] The term used to describe runaway slaves, "maroon," derived from the Spanish term, "cimarron," "a domesticated animal that had reverted back to a wild state."[28] Daily accounts confirm that the loss of animal life from disease was as important as the death of slaves from illness or accident. Noting the duties of the plantation manager, Ducoeurjoly advised that a journal be kept to record "the birth and death of the slaves, and domestic animals."[29] Laborie concurred: "The journal must contain a state of the negroes and cattle, a state of the births and deaths."[30] Overseers used the same types of restraints, such as collars, on slaves that were employed on animals. Whips struck the backs of both human and nonhuman creatures. The increasing use of slaves as objects of scientific study and experimentation doomed men and women to the inquiring gaze of the physician and the naturalist in Saint Domingue. Scientists argued that slaves, like animals, experienced little or no pain.

In order to support their labor system, slaveholders made frequent reference to the similarities that they perceived to exist between slaves and animals. Abolitionists, likewise, stressed the "logic of domination" to advance their cause. Abolitionists accused slaveowners of treating their slaves inhumanely, and their appeals to end slavery emphasized that slavery muddled the distinction between human and animal.[31]

The animalization of human beings not only supported Saint Domingue's slave system but also sustained the racial divisions that existed in the colony. Theorists separated men and women into racial categories whose names were taken from the animal kingdom; Moreau de Saint-Méry's racial chart referred to biracial residents as marabou, a bird, and griffin, a type of dog.[32] Commentators described the inferior economic and social positions held by the *Mésalliés*, or white men who married women of color, and the prevalence of concubinage in animalistic terms. Dutertre believed that such relationships were associations between different species and the children who resulted from them were aberrations. In fact, *mulatto*, a term of sixteenth-century Spanish origin, is derived etymologically from "mule," a sterile creature produced by a horse and an ass. The sterility ascribed to women of color may even have been founded upon this notion.[33]

Saint Domingue and the Medical Care of Animals

The colonists of Saint Domingue recognized the significant roles that animals played in colonial history, economy, and slave culture. As a result, keeping animals healthy was a high priority. Planters and their employees feared epizootics, or outbreaks of animal diseases. Moreau de Saint-Méry noted that animals were "difficult to replace and the existence of which becomes each day more uncertain by epizootics."[34] Epizootics were common occurrences; draft animals such as mules suffered from various illnesses, including *morve*, or glanders.[35] Horses and sheep also fell victim to disease, most especially anthrax. These epizootics not only endangered animal life but had the potential to destroy human life, especially the lives of individuals who came in contact with nonhuman creatures. On the plantations, those individuals were slaves, an expensive labor source. Both anthrax and glanders were extremely dangerous to the human population. When glanders attacked enslaved men and women, it was likely confused with yaws from the similar symptoms, such as nodular eruptions on the face, arms, and legs.[36]

Colonial officials used legal means in order to curb the spread of animal disease. In November 1750, for instance, they passed an ordinance to prevent the spread of an epizootic that was killing horses in the Cul-de-Sac region. They instructed three physicians, two of whom were royally appointed, to remain in the area to offer assistance. They also ordered soldiers to stop the removal of animals from the region as well as the entry of creatures from outside areas, and they commanded the soldiers to make daily and nightly excursions on horseback in order to force residents to bury dead animals. If coercion did not succeed in convincing inhabitants to inter dead animals, the law threatened owners with monetary fines. The epizootic finally ended in January 1751 with the death of more than 1,000 horses. Unfortunately, in 1752, another epizootic raged; it was so severe that the local government was unable to conduct business and postponed its meeting until the following January.[37]

In addition to epizootics of glanders and anthrax, outbreaks of rabies also frightened residents of Saint Domingue and threatened livestock as well as slaves. According to legal documents, the disease was rarely seen in the colony prior to the 1760s, the period when many colonists reported that rabies appeared in the towns and on the plantations. In March 1762 the *Conseil* of the Cap implemented measures designed to arrest the transmission of the disease. Lawmakers urged physicians and surgeons to make known the names of the victims of the disease and publish the remedies employed. In addition, townspeople were ordered to destroy dogs, and rural residents were told to restrain healthy canines and exterminate and burn those that appeared to be infected.[38] In September of the same year, citizens of Port-au-Prince reported that rabid dogs stalked the streets of the city, biting and killing Europeans, Creoles, free blacks, and slaves. Lawmakers instructed the inhabitants to kill, drown if necessary, their dogs within twenty-four hours of the decree being published.[39]

The frequency of legislation that concentrated on veterinary issues increased after 1762, the year when veterinary schools were established in France, one at Lyons and one in Alfort. These schools were reactions to the call for better equine medicine (warfare depended on the ability of a nation to field healthy horses) and to the anxiety created by the loss of livestock as a result of epizootics.[40] After receiving royal permission, Claude Bourgelat, a self-taught veterinary surgeon, opened the school in Lyons in 1762 and left one year later in order to take charge of the school at Alfort, an institution established by another well-known animal care practitioner and veterinary author and educator, Philippe-Étienne LaFosse.[41]

Professional veterinary care came to Saint Domingue two decades after its appearance in France. To deal with epizootics, the Saint Domingue government, in 1782, hired two official or royal veterinarians, Dutilleul and Gelin, both of whom were trained in French veterinary schools. At the urging of satisfied customers, colonial officials also awarded an honorary degree to Jean LaPole, a self-taught veterinarian. Moreau de Saint-Méry recorded that a Monsieur de Boynes contracted with the veterinary school in Alfort, France, to provide students to reside and practice in the French colonies for twelve years. De Boynes believed that veterinarians were useful subjects of a colony where the price of animals was so dear and where it was difficult to replace animals lost to disease.[42]

Plantation managers and absentee landowners agreed with de Boynes's assessment. Correspondence between proprietors and their employees are filled with references to animals dead from epizootics and the actions taken to prevent further loss of animal life. From July 1789 to April 1790 worries over an epizootic occupied the mind of LeCesne and the letters that he wrote to his employers. On 16 July 1789 he briefly alluded to "the epidemic that is ravaging the animals in the area. . . . I have learned . . . that the malady is very contagious." After consulting with a veterinarian, he reported in August that "The veterinarian assures me that with the first drops of rain, the epidemic will disappear. As this sickness appears to be an inflammation occasioned by the heat, I have not failed to bathe all your animals two and often three times a day." LeCesne wanted to reassure his employers that all possible measures were being taken to prevent an outbreak of the disease. By November, his efforts had failed, and both mules and cattle were under attack. In early 1790 he recorded that "What is even more frightening still is that men, especially slaves, are subject to it and have already been its victims." LeCesne mentioned that he eagerly sought out any information about the epidemic and took the precautions advised by the "veterinary artists" in the newspapers. The recommendations of these *artistes vétérinaires*, however, disappointed LeCesne and his neighbors. Attempting to deflect any criticism from his employers on the way he had handled the problem, he said that the losses that the planters sustained were "the fault of veterinary artists, who are true charlatans, promising to cure this illness." His letter of 8 April finally brought good news—the epizootic had ended.[43]

The *Cercle des Philadelphes*, Saint Domingue's scientific and medical society, also concerned itself with veterinary medicine and education through the publication of *Recherches, Mémoires et Observations sur les Maladies Épizootiques de Saint-Domingue*. The members provided numerous accounts of epizootics that ravaged herds of mules and cattle. One of the contributors, Monsieur Darnaudin, encouraged royal physicians and surgeons as well as veterinarians to perform their official duties by visiting warehouses and plantations where epizootics existed, by examining animals, and by suggesting the best ways for stopping the progress of disease.

Popular Practitioners of Veterinary Medicine

Because professional veterinarians were few in number, the importance of livestock to the economy of Saint Domingue, the European tradition of consulting popular practitioners of animal medicine, and the isolation that characterized much of Saint Domingue, plantation managers turned to veterinary manuals, plantation surgeons, and slaves for veterinary assistance. Planters, their employees, plantations surgeons, and slaves treated nonhuman and human animals and used a variety of techniques and remedies to prevent outbreaks of disease and to deal with epidemics.

Just as they employed traditional European therapies to deal with human disease, planters and their employees utilized known recipes and herbs to treat animal ailments. LeCesne, for instance, noted repeatedly that he made sure to nourish and bathe the animals under his authority in order to prevent the outbreak of disease. When common techniques failed them, they often turned to veterinary manuals for advice. Guides written for farriers, grooms, and horse owners were quite popular in Europe, and they made their way to Saint Domingue. In his manual on how to establish a productive coffee plantation, Laborie mentioned *Our Perfect Farmer* and *Rustic House* as useful texts for understanding how to deal with common animal illnesses, wounds, and accidents.[44]

If their own ministrations failed, planters and their managers often called upon plantation surgeons, who not only treated human patients but also turned their attention to animals when a qualified veterinarian was unavailable. LeCesne depended on the plantation surgeon Danger during epizootics. When illness devastated the plantation's mule population, Danger performed surgery on the creatures and recommended treatments that LeCesne might use to prevent additional loss of animal life.[45]

Slaves employed as *gardiens de bêtes,* or animal caretakers, practiced veterinary medicine too. Like other forms of plantation labor, animal caretaking had a gendered component. Female slaves generally looked after poultry, sheep, and goats, while men watched over larger draft animals.[46] Laborie gave an excellent example of the gendered division of work when he stated, "The Driver, or Chief of the Negroes and Mules, employed in carriage, should be faithful and attentive to the care and good plight of his beasts. He ought to know to cure their wounds and ordinary distempers."[47] Laborie's statement demonstrated that some slaves were veterinary specialists because of the care they provided to certain creatures. The gendering of animal care labor can be traced to the tendency to identify animals as either masculine or feminine. Animals that were smaller and more subject to confinement were the responsibility of women, while larger and stronger creatures, such as horses, mules, and cattle, came under the authority of male slaves.[48] Women's care of chickens, for example, emerged from the gender symbolism ascribed to the nonhuman creatures. In European lore, the hen represented the best qualities of motherhood. Classical authors praised her instinct to nurture her young and protect them from harm. The egg she produced also had powerful connotations. It represented fertility, birth, and renewal.[49]

Caring for animals by enslaved men and women also was affected by the way in which animals were represented, understood, and tended in Africa. Africans whose local economies depended on cattle became valuable commodities in the slave trade. In particular, slaves from Senegambia were experienced in tending livestock.[50]

The skills of the enslaved veterinary artists had several sources. They learned about veterinary therapies in Africa or via knowledge passed down from an elder African slave. For centuries, African herdsmen and women as well as healers of animals (who also treated humans) ministered to ailing animals. Veterinary knowledge derived from both family tradition and practical experience. Causes of animal disease were attributed to natural and supernatural forces. Treatment procedures include herbal remedies, inoculation, surgery, and rituals such as purification ceremonies.[51] In addition to their knowledge of traditional African veterinary therapies, animal caretakers improvised with plants available in Saint Domingue. Like African veterinary practitioners, they likely observed the plants that ailing animals ate and then experimented with the plants.[52] In many cases, animal by-products also were employed as remedies. Animal products constituted the pharmacopeias of various medical systems, including those of Africa and Europe. Animals and their derivatives such as eggs, honey, and dung not only figured into drug therapy but also were employed to ward off disastrous environmental events and to divine and change future occurrences. Finally, some slaves were taught veterinary medical skills by masters who were veterinary specialists themselves. In 1781 Sieur Furgeot, an expert farrier who lived in Cap-François, advertised the sale of an enslaved man who knew how "to dress wounds, both human and animal, superlatively." The slaveowner also offered for sale a forge with accompanying instruments and a collection of medicines for both human and animal use.[53]

Slaveowners and plantation managers consulted *gardiens de bêtes* when animals were victims of epizootics. The well-educated *Cercle des Philadelphes* also was interested in their work and noted the remedies they employed. These members mentioned that animal caretakers worked in hospitals built solely for the care of sick animals and generally employed frictions (remedies rubbed on the skin). Similarly, Laborie wrote, "A little separate stable is . . . necessary in another place, but within reach, for the animals which have contagious distempers."[54] The work of the *gardiens de bêtes* was very dangerous because of diseases that spread from animals to their caretakers. One of the contributors to the *Cercle des Philadelphes* book, Monsieur Darnaudin, recorded the case of a *gardeur des animaux malades* (enslaved caretaker of sick animals) who he believed contracted an illness from diseased animals and died.[55]

The choice of a *gardien de bêtes* was an important decision for the manager or planter to make. The animal caretaker had authority over and the care of very significant plantation commodities. Contributors to the *Cercle des Philadelphes* text on epizootics noted that the job of conducting the animals to pastureland generally was given to young slave boys, a responsibility that young boys in Europe also held. Similarly, Ducoeurjoly said that slaves who were not physically robust usually were chosen to care for the animals. Laborie noted, "In general, an estate has people set apart for keeping of cattle; but if the negroes employed on this duty are not changed every week, they become idle and licentious."[56] Members of the *Cercle des Philadelphes* encouraged planters to abandon these practices and ensure that only the most intelligent slaves were given charge of animals.[57] The author of an article on the difficulties of raising livestock in Saint Domingue blamed slaves for the high death rates among animals. He claimed that "many slaves do not understand the illnesses to which horned beasts are subject nor how to remedy them."[58] The negative assessment of the *gardiens de bête* by these writers may, however, have been inaccurate. The records compiled by LeCesne, for example, noted that his animal caretakers were men of good health: Philippon, a twenty-nine-year-old African slave who cared for cattle, and Simon, a twenty-nine-year-old Creole slave who was responsible for mules.[59] Similarly, accounts from the Chavanne plantation note that a thirty-year-old man named Mathieu held the title of *gardien d'animaux*. Mathieu most likely was responsible for the animals involved in the production of sugar. Because of his skills, this enslaved man was the second most valuable slave on the plantation; only the commander was worth more money. This plantation also possessed an enslaved man, twenty-two-year-old Adonis, who cared for cattle, and four preteen boys who watched over the mules and cattle.[60]

Pacotilleurs, or peddlers, also provided veterinary treatment on the plantations. Slaves, free blacks, and *libres de fait* worked as *pacotilleurs,* selling small European-made items and baubles throughout the slave quarters, practicing medicine, and offering veterinary therapies. Because of their ability to travel all over the slave quarters and between plantations, peddlers posed two significant risks to white planters: They were possible transmitters of disease because of their itinerant work and were sources of rebellion.[61] Laborie counseled: "I observe that hawkers ought to be cautiously admitted into estates, and never be permitted to enter into, or stay, in the *negroe* houses. They are often retailers of corruption, and promoters of bad inclinations."[62]

Whites also eyed *gardiens de bêtes* suspiciously. Élie Monnereau, who wrote a manual on how to run a profitable indigo plantation, warned would-be proprietors that the *gardiens de bêtes* often participated in schemes to steal or destroy plantation livestock.[63] Like many other types of enslaved healers, the *gardiens de bêtes* held high-ranking positions within the slave hierarchy, but their considerable status made their masters suspicious of them. Descriptions of animal caretakers often portrayed them as loners who possessed ample time to ponder their existence. Whites construed their knowledge of herbs as the power to harm as well as heal. The life and influence of a *gardien de bête* named Makandal and his association with the *pacotilleurs* indicate that the whites were correct in placing great importance on the choice of the *gardien de bêtes* and in fearing the peddlers. Through his life and work, Makandal inspired his fellow slaves to throw off the chains of slavery and gain their freedom.

The History of Makandal

Makandal was a prized African-born slave held in high esteem by his master, a man named Le Normand de Mézy. According to a newspaper account, he had learned how to read and write the Arabic language and how to practice herbalism and medicine in Africa. The author recounted, "He possessed great knowledge of the medicine of his country and the efficacy of medicinal plants."[64] As we have seen, herbalism was a significant component of West African medical care. Some of Makandal's contemporaries believed he might have been a Muslim because of reports that he invoked the name of Allah.[65] These reports and Makandal's familiarity with the Arabic language might mean that he adhered to Islam. If so, his use of herbal medicine might have come from his Islamic background. At the very least, he appeared to be familiar with Islamic medicine. Koranic teachers provided medical care by diagnosing and attending to sicknesses brought about by natural and supernatural causes and by supplying talismans or charms. Islamic medicine in West Africa not only incorporated healing herbs but also emphasized the medicine of the Prophet (deeds, sayings, and anecdotes of Muhammad that dealt with medical care), the numerical healing power of Koranic verses, the names of religious figures such as angels, prophets, and saints, magic, and divination.[66] In addition, some Muslims believed that *jinn,* or genies that assume human or animal forms, were responsible for supernatural causes of illness and accepted the idea that *shetani,* or spirits, possessed human beings and brought about sickness.[67]

Makandal's ability to treat illnesses deemed incurable by French and Creole doctors made him a favorite among his fellow slaves, who often sent for him in order to ask him to send a leaf or root that would bring them good health. Makandal's abilities as a healer may have assisted him in his work as *gardien de bêtes,* a position he held after having lost his hand in a work accident. Despite his high status (or perhaps because of it), Makandal ran away from the plantation and escaped to the mountains of Saint Domingue. A love affair with a fellow slave and physical violence at the hands of his master convinced him to abscond.[68]

During his time as a fugitive, Makandal became a legendary figure. His story cannot be separated from the history of the maroons and the powerful influence that they had on maintaining and fostering resistance that led to the revolution in Haiti. Maroons, or runaway slaves, chose to remove themselves from slavery in many ways. Advertisements seeking the return of runaway slaves were common sights in colonial newspapers.[69] Some slaves practiced *petit marronnage:* They ran away from their masters for short periods of time and lived on the outskirts of the plantations. Other slaves participated in *grand marronnage:* They permanently escaped to urban areas, to the border areas that separated French and Spanish Saint Domingue, or, like Makandal, to the mountains.[70]

In the mountains, Makandal assumed authority over a network of agents throughout the colony. Makandal's associates were the *pacotilleurs* who went about the plantations, bringing poisoned fruits to the men and women Makandal had chosen for death. According to one report, his recruitment of enslaved followers was astounding—some plantations lost as many as 90 percent of newly purchased slaves.[71] Reportedly, his vast network of followers would murder at his command. In addition to killing slaves and whites, Makandal and the *pacotilleurs* also poisoned animals. By targeting slaves and animals, they hoped to damage plantation productivity and the colonial economy. The choice of slaves as prey also shows that Makandal had appropriated the European tendency to equate slaves with nonhuman animals. Moreover, by eliminating slaves, he and his followers could coerce allegiance through terrorism. Ultimately, Makandal hoped to advance to the annihilation of whites. He asserted that the African gods had called him to be a *papalwa* (high priest) who would lead his children back to the African homeland. Slaves believed he had supernatural powers; he reportedly fashioned fetishes out of wood, which he claimed talked to him and told him who would die. In the words of Moreau de Saint Méry, Makandal's greatest plan was "to eradicate from the face of the earth all those who were not black."[72] In order to accomplish this feat, he planned to poison the water supply of Cap-François, one of Saint Domingue's largest cities. Makandal's immediate goal was not realized; tipped off by a young slave boy, white residents apprehended him at a *calenda* (dance) at the Dufresne plantation in the parish of Limbé. His capture there was short-lived; assisted by his supporters, he escaped from the house in which he was being confined and fled. Caught a short time later and brought to justice, Makandal was condemned in 1758 to be burned alive in Cap-François. Among the accusations rendered against him was the charge that he formulated and sold magical packets and poisons to blacks. He was executed and his ashes were scattered to the wind, but not before striking terror as well as inspiring hope in the hearts of his fellow slaves. In the midst of the fire, Makandal strained against the cords that held him and broke free. The slaves assembled cried out, "Makandal is saved! Makandal is saved!" Not to be foiled, colonial officials grabbed hold of him, tied him once again, and threw him into the fire. Claiming to be able to transform himself into various creatures, Makandal declared that he would take the shape of a fly in order to escape from the flames. Many slaves took him at his word; they believed he had simply flown away.[73]

The Legend of Makandal and the Haitian Revolution

Even though Makandal's body was burned, his spirit and ideology smoldered for decades, even centuries. Makandal and his followers initiated and implemented an ideology of resistance via occupational sabotage and the destruction of human and animal life. Just as the tale of the *boucanier* became the founding myth for French residents of the Caribbean, the story of Makandal became the basis for stories of revolutionary struggle in Saint Domingue and eventually throughout the Caribbean.

The legend of Makandal grew swiftly after his death. He became immortalized in art, literature, oral history, and law. A likeness of him and three of his accomplices was painted and sent to France; Moreau de Saint-Méry eventually purchased it. The lead character in a London play, a rebellious slave, was named Makandal.[74] Literary accounts of slaves using poison and poisonous plants as weapons drew from Makandal's history. Such stories told of slaves trained in Africa who used plants to destroy slaves (even members of their own families), animals, and eventually whites. Ducoeurjoly mentioned that most often these slaves, like Makandal, were high-ranking and beloved by their masters.[75] He chose to highlight this fact in order to caution slaveholders from relaxing their authority over slaves. Whispering his name and recounting his deeds, slaves continued to support and push forward Makandal's revolutionary dreams. He became a member of the pantheon of gods worshiped by the practitioners of vodou.[76] His name, a Kongo word for amulet, became synonymous with his followers, the packets they produced and sold, and the poisons they distributed, all referred to as *macandals*.[77] The terror that Makandal inspired also was evident in the proliferation of laws that attempted to curb the distribution of poisons, the circulation of medical remedies by slaves, and the movement of slaves from one area to another. In the same year as his capture and execution, the *Conseil* of the Cap prohibited slaves from making or selling the so-called packets. They based this prohibition on a 1682 law that forbade the distribution of profane materials. This ordinance also ordered slaveowners to strictly supervise slaves like herbalists and *hospitalières* who distributed medical remedies to other slaves.[78] In April 1758 the *Conseil* attempted to curb the mobility of the *pacotilleurs* by prohibiting slaves, even with permission from their masters, from selling merchandise, including sugar, sugarcane, coffee, and manufactured utensils at the markets or at particular homes.[79]

The scandal generated by Makandal prompted an intellectual *cause célèbre,* and authors weighed in on the controversy—was poisoning, like that undertaken by Makandal, a significant threat? Many writers answered with a resounding yes. Dazille argued that poisoning was an outcome of the institution of slavery. He saw Saint Domingue as "a nation where the free man and the enslaved man cultivate the same earth, where one has without end to dread the effects of power, and the other those of vengeance." Because slavery engendered such emotions, he believed it necessary for men of medicine to "know how to distinguish the effects of poison from those that accompany the maladies to which humanity is exposed without cease."[80] Bertin said that slaves possessed knowledge of herbal poisons, but that they tended to use toxins they stole from their masters. The herbal poisons consisted of certain roots that left black spots on the tongues of the victims and the sap of the Manchineel tree, which caused death by attacking the stomach and lungs. Toxins that they gained from their masters usually included arsenic.[81]

The majority of physicians, however, opposed the idea that illness was the result of poisoning committed by the slaves. Whether a treatise dealt with human diseases or animal affliction, learned men argued that sickness was, by and large, due to physical factors, such as weather or poor nutrition. They maintained that the contrary view was a misperception on the part of ignorant whites and their unskilled European medical caretakers.[82]

Lay commentators, likewise, had their own opinions on whether slaves participated in poisonings. Girod-Chantrans believed that jealousy drove black men to kill other slaves and even to murder their masters. He asserted that jealousy was simply part of their nature. The sexual liberties that masters and other slaves took with the female slaves enraged male slaves and made them commit murder. Girod-Chantrans said that the slaves killed their fellow bondsmen by offering them poisoned mixtures of herbs and greens. He also claimed that male slaves turned the masters' toxins on the masters themselves.[83]

Hilliard d'Auberteuil said that if slaves poisoned, these acts were rare and were perpetrated by means of venoms stolen from slaveholders. He declared, "If the slaves were naturally wicked, a single man would not govern a hundred slaves in the middle of the woods, on a remote mountain, as has been the practice for one hundred years. The master lives safely surrounded by his atelier and his domestics and is able to give them arms without dreading that they will be turned against him."[84] Moreau de Saint-Méry, likewise, doubted that slaves engaged in poisoning against their masters. He attributed most illnesses to physical and climatic causes, while admitting that self-professing sorcerers among the African slaves existed.[85]

The fear that Makandal and his fellow slaves created led to a violent backlash against slaves suspected of poisoning. In 1758, the same year that Makandal was executed, three other slaves named Samba, Colas, and Lafleur were imprisoned and awaited execution on charges of poisoning. The circumstances of their being put to death reflected the animalization of enslaved men and women that had taken place over the course of several centuries. Several physicians, including Lacq, *médecin du Roi*, Daubenton, Boyer, Allies, Pagès, and Keau, had the authority to experiment on the men with drugs suspected of being used as poisons by the slaves. After conducting an experiment, they reported, "having given to a slave an emulsion made with a half-ounce of a seed common in America. After one hour, the slave was immobile, unconscious, having a thick tongue, sticky saliva, a yellowish mucous in the nose."[86] As a result of the experiments, two of the slaves died.[87]

Despite the attempt by colonial authorities to stop the poisoning, legal records demonstrate that it continued for decades. In 1765 a wave of poisonings rocked La Sucrerie Cottineau. Not only were animals killed, but very valuable slaves, the *sucriers* (slaves involved in sugar refining), were being murdered. The absentee planters advised the manager to inspect the nostrils of animals because slaves killed the creatures by inserting pointed sticks laced with poison into the orifices. Using all means necessary to get to the bottom of the mystery, the manager finally put a stop to the poisonings by making the animal caretakers responsible for the deaths. Despite the manager's investigations, the killing of slaves continued; seven slaves were eventually executed and one was imprisoned for the crimes.[88] In the late 1770s the *Conseil* of Cap-François condemned a slave named Jacques to be burned alive after having been found to possess a container of arsenic and to have poisoned 100 animals belonging to his master over the course of eight months. Based on his crimes, Jacques may have been a *pacotilleur* who traveled across his master's plantation and between it and others, selling poisons and destroying animals.[89] At the Fleuriau plantation, three house slaves plotted to poison whites; they succeeded in killing an attorney named Rasseteau. Their plan to murder the manager, however, did not succeed. The poison that M. Leremboura was intended to ingest was fed to a dog, which died immediately. Like Jacques, the enslaved men were imprisoned awaiting execution.[90]

Although actual poisonings took place, accidental and natural cases of poisoning helped to feed the legend of Makandal and keep it alive for decades. Saint Domingue was an environment that presented natural poisoning dangers. Poisonous snakes and crabs proliferated, residents faced death if they consumed toxic sardines, and people could easily obtain and eat poisonous fruit. The remedies the slaves used did have potentially fatal side effects if they were administered incorrectly. The castor oil plant, for example, provided castor oil, a remedy that served many beneficial purposes, but a single castor bean, if ingested, causes death. African healers were also limited by the ecology of Saint Domingue, which differed from that of the Old World. It is not unreasonable to imagine that healers might mistakenly use a Saint Domingue plant that was similar in appearance but not in purpose to one with which they had been familiar in Africa.[91] Finally, illnesses that struck slaves, animals, and members of the planter family were often attributed to poisoning. When an enslaved healer was consulted and the patient died, it was easy to blame the slave practitioner. Charges of poisoning leveled against the *pacotilleurs* may even have emerged from unsuccessful medical or veterinary treatments that they had provided.

Ultimately, enslaved men and women created a revolutionary identity from Makandal's life and legend. They chose Makandal, the introspective and intelligent *gardien de bêtes,* as their mythic hero. The myth of Makandal influenced events associated with the Haitian Revolution, shaped the history of the greatest revolutionary leader in Saint Domingue, Toussaint-Louverture, and inspired other Caribbean radicals. The location for organizing one of the most important slave rebellions of the Haitian Revolution took place only ten miles from Makandal's home as a slave, the plantation of Le Normand de Mézy. On Sunday, 14 August 1791, a group of high-ranking slaves met in order to discuss plans to foment a rebellion. The main participants were coachmen, or enslaved men who cared for their masters' horses and who had the opportunity to travel widely because they had access to transportation. A slave later revealed that "all drivers, coachmen, domestics and confidential negroes . . . formed a plot to set fire to the plantations and murder all the whites."[92] One week later, slaves gathered and participated in the Bois-Caiman vodou ceremony on 21 August 1791.[93] Was the spirit of Makandal whirling in their minds and on their lips? It likely was. The leader of the ceremony, Boukman, was, like Makandal, a revered figure; he also was his master's coachman.[94] After Boukman sacrificed a pig, those in attendance drank its blood and took its hairs as talismans that would protect them from harm. Like Makandal's *pacotilleurs,* the associates of Boukman pledged their allegiance to him. Two days after the ceremony, slaves set fire to a neighboring plantation. Their plot was not only to torch the one plantation, but to immolate adjacent landholdings. A week later, the slave rebellion of 1791 was underway.[95]

But Makandal's influence on the Haitian Revolution did not stop there. The mythology that surrounded Makandal became incorporated into the life and legend of Haiti's greatest leader, Toussaint-Louverture. Historians have acknowledged the difficulty in coming to know the real Toussaint; like Makandal's life story, it is hard to separate Toussaint's history from his hagiography. Toussaint may have knowingly played upon his association with Makandal; two biographies of Toussaint emphasize his cunningness and ability to manipulate his supporters as well as his detractors.[96] Reportedly, at the age of thirteen, Toussaint-Louverture witnessed the burning of Makandal and vowed to bring Makandal's dream to fruition. In his teens, Toussaint, like Makandal, held the position of *gardien de bêtes,* taking care of the cattle on his master's plantation. Histories of the great leader of the Haitian Revolution emphasize that his position as caretaker to his master's nonhuman creatures gave him the freedom and time alone to consider his plight and the cruelty that he witnessed daily. His work also demonstrated his familiarity with remedies that could be used to protect his animal charges as well as the slaves who journeyed to his doorstep for assistance. Like Makandal, his skill with medicinal plants came from his African background; his father taught him how to identify and employ herbs. Finally, the high status and respect that his labor afforded him meant that his fellow slaves saw in him a leader to be followed. According to one of his contemporaries, General François Marie de Kerversau, Toussaint-Louverture was "respected by the Africans as a sort of Makandal."[97] Reportedly, his own master recognized his skills and promoted him from a simple guardian of animals to the caretaker of his prized horses. His emancipation from slavery in 1776 did not quench his desire to help his brothers and sisters in bondage; by 1793 he embraced and spoke openly about the notion of general emancipation. Allegedly, his military career started with his service as an herbalist to the guerilla troops of Jean-François.[98] The identification of Toussaint-Louverture with Makandal became so great that one of Toussaint's foremost modern biographers, Pierre Pluchon, described him as "a Catholic Makandal" who "relied on the power of faith and magical ideas" to bolster his authority and the allegiance of his followers.[99]

Makandal also inspired Jean-Jacques Dessalines, the former slave and Haitian revolutionary who eventually became the first emperor of Haiti. Dessalines routinely consulted *macandalistes* and used their techniques in order to determine the loyalty of particular individuals. Like the followers of Makandal, Dessalines judged the intentions of a person by assessing the humidity or dryness of the tobacco contained in his snuffbox. Dessalines also used sorcery in order to make himself invisible so that he could inspect French camps and cross through enemy lines to speak with his soldiers. He encouraged his troops by telling them that their deaths on the battlefield would result in their transportation to Africa, where they would be reunited with their leader, Toussaint-Louverture. The connection between Haitian revolutionaries like Dessalines and Makandal is so enduring that Haitian oral tradition includes songs in which Dessalines is praised for bringing new magic to the Haitian people and in which Makandal warns Dessalines to stay away from Pont-Rouge, the site of Dessalines's brutal death.[100]

Famous as well as unknown men and women both in Saint Domingue and in neighboring islands worked to bring Makandal's vision to life. During the Haitian Revolution, a group of enslaved women successfully implemented Makandal's plot to murder whites by poisoning a water supply with copper utensils dumped into a well. After drinking the water, many soldiers died.[101] In 1791 a peddler in Jamaica named Milburn's Jack followed the lead of Makandal's *pacotilleurs* by using his trading network to gain supplies of gunpowder with which to resist the island's masters. The inspiration provided by Makandal and the *pacotilleurs* was not lost on an administrative assembly, which commented on the dangers that a vast network of peddlers led by a charismatic leader might pose.[102]

Conclusion

Enslaved veterinary practitioners and the animals for which they cared were crucial actors in the colonial and revolutionary dramas that unfolded in eighteenth-century Saint Domingue. Their coerced labor contributed to the development of one of France's most productive and wealthiest colonies. Enslaved veterinary artists provided expense-free medical care to both human and nonhuman animals. Most important, slave veterinarians and their animal charges served as important symbols throughout the colony's history. European and Creole settlers embraced the image of the *boucanier* to highlight their predatory power over both animals and slaves. The slave system on which the colony was built depended upon the animalization of African men and women. Enslaved men and women, on the other hand, chose the figure of the introspective and intelligent *gardien de bêtes*, personified by Makandal and eventually Toussaint-Louverture, as the leader of their revolution and the founder of a free Haiti.

6 Magnetism in Eighteenth-Century Saint Domingue: The Case of the Enslaved Magnetists and Their Fight for Freedom

> Later Mesmer boasted that the new republic—now called Haiti—owed its independence to him.
>
> —Henri F. Ellenberger, 1970

The last quarter of the eighteenth century was a tumultuous period in the history of French medicine. Official practitioners clashed with one another and against the so-called medical mountebanks. In France, the most famous episodes in this era of medical agitation were the rise and swift descent of mesmerism. Historians have interpreted the backlash against mesmerism as the assertion of academic, privileged physic in the face of revolutionary medicine; as the affirmation of the political, social, and moral status quo through a critique of the relationship between the male magnetizer and the female patient; and as the development of modern psychiatry.[1] A mesmerist, or magnetist, controversy, led by enslaved mesmerists, likewise existed in Saint Domingue.[2] The arrest and subsequent punishment of the slave magnetizers were attacks on the healing undertaken by slaves and people of color as well as assaults on slaves who dared to oppose the white population. White residents saw mesmerist activity as a form of resistance and did everything in their power to eliminate it. In Haiti mesmerism became synonymous with freedom. For its supporters, magnetism offered freedom from established medicine, but, what is more significant, freedom from the authority of the white master; to its detractors, mesmerism's promise of freedom signified the dangerous breakdown of hierarchy, the deterioration of social position, and, what was most frightening, the potential destruction of Saint Domingue's slave society.

The History of Mesmerism in Europe

In the 1780s Anton Mesmer and his disciples held France in a trance. After arriving in Paris in 1778, Mesmer, a university-educated German physician, declared that a superfine liquid existed everywhere and that he was able to harness its power by means of specially built tubs. This power, termed mesmerism and comparable to the effects of "animal magnetism," reportedly cured numerous ailments, including smallpox, cancer, gout, jaundice, ulcers, and hernia. Members of the Parisian *beau monde* flocked to witness and participate in mesmerist treatments. Mesmer's patients and supporters included court aristocrats, wealthy commoners, members of the Paris Parlement, and some paupers whom Mesmer graciously and shrewdly treated for free. In his apartments, they would find Mesmer, a metal wand in hand, welcoming them and directing them to the *baquet*, or wooden tub. Once assembled, his clients took hold of iron rods attached to the tub and joined fingers. A rope bound the group together as one. During the mesmerist treatment, crises, including convulsions, yawning, laughter, crying, fainting, evacuations, and expectorations, occurred and signaled the restoration of the body's natural balance. Disease, or the blockage of superfine liquid or fluid within the body, had ended and the body was returned to health.[3]

Mesmerism appealed to men and women of the eighteenth century because it was not dissimilar to ancient medical notions that attributed disease to an imbalance, deficiency, or excess of a particular humor or fluid. Moreover, Mesmer's personal touch (his operations included massage), communal healing, and flair for the dramatic pleased patients who were used to the ministrations of aloof physicians who offered aggressive remedies like bloodletting and purges in the dark stillness of the sickroom. Mesmer was more like the mountebanks who entertained the crowds from the backs of carriages or in the marketplaces. Furthermore, his performances echoed the royal rituals of the sacred touch. Mesmer's magnetism also resonated with consumers of Enlightenment popular science. Gravitation, electricity, ballooning, and magnetic energy—all were in the air and discussed at common cafés and posh salons. Finally, the master's audience welcomed his timely talk of perfection in both the medical and moral universes.[4]

Mesmer profited handsomely from his technique; his annual income stood at approximately 96,000 *livres* while his expenses totaled around 20,000 *livres*. The establishment of the Society of Harmony in 1783 provided Mesmer with forty-eight pupils who paid 2,400 *livres* to receive instruction from the master.[5] But the miraculous recoveries recorded round the tubs and the money made from them provoked skeptical responses from the French medical, scientific, and political establishment. In 1784 the Crown appointed two commissions to investigate mesmerism. Members of the Paris faculty of medicine and the Academy of Sciences, including significant medical and scientific authorities like Antoine Laurent Lavoisier, Joseph Ignace Guillotine, and Benjamin Franklin, made up the first commission, while the other consisted of members of the Royal Society of Medicine. Both groups condemned mesmerism. Attacking it at its healing source, the members reported that the universal liquid did not exist. Despite their Enlightenment dream that medicine would someday alleviate the ills of society, the commissioners realized that the joyous day had not yet arrived. Adopting a paternalistic air, they concluded that mesmerist therapies offered false hope for the suffering. They also asserted that purported cures were nothing more than fantasies that stemmed only from the overactive imaginations of patients, many of whom were women. The spokesmen, moreover, refuted Mesmer's claim of the unity between humanity and the rest of creation. Humanity, more specifically rational man, reigned over God's lesser creatures, both human and non-human. Above all, the commissioners feared Mesmer's disruption of the medical, moral, and political orders. The ability of the fluid and Mesmer to transcend class boundaries put the hierarchical nature of French society, including its medical component, in jeopardy. The physical agitation that characterized mesmerist treatment, especially the convulsions to which his female patients were subject, threatened morality through its potential to unleash sexual excess and libertinage. In order to protect the French Crown, women, men, and medicine—mesmerism had to stop.[6]

Mesmer and his followers vigorously fought the commissions' conclusions. According to the mesmerists, mainstream medicine was deadly and unnatural; it offered dangerous remedies that opposed the guiding hand of nature. In addition, medicine, like the state, profited from the suffering of men and women. By condemning Mesmer and his work, official medical practitioners revealed that they were not interested in easing the pain of humanity; Mesmer, on the other hand, had the good of the people in mind. He argued that his techniques brought men and women of all social classes together; physicians and other members of the medical corpus were intent on keeping them separated. A hierarchal society echoed the corporate structure of eighteenth-century medicine. Finally, Mesmer and his associates rejected the commissions' accusations that the patient's imagination prompted the physical expression of mesmerist cures, and the mesmerists downplayed the convulsions of their female clients.[7]

In spite of the attack on mesmerism in the French capital, the theory and the practices associated with it enjoyed widespread appeal in the French provinces. In fact, residents of the provinces were the main supporters of the movement from 1786 to 1789. Mesmer's tour of southern France aided his cause. Famous disciples like the Marquis de Puységur, Armand-Marie-Jacques de Chastenet, also assisted in spreading the mesmerist gospel outside Paris. In the provinces, town leaders, including prominent doctors, soldiers, priests, and government officials, accepted and promoted mesmerism. The ambivalence of the provincial press and the lax attitude of police instructed to ferret out what some provincial critics described as yet another form of charlatanism also contributed to the reign of mesmerism in the French countryside and provincial cities.[8]

Mesmerism in Saint Domingue

Seventeen eighty-four was an important year for mesmerism. In the French metropole, animal magnetism came under official censure. It remained, however, a popular pursuit in the French provinces. Further away, in the French colony of Saint Domingue, mesmerism enjoyed widespread appeal, especially among the upper strata of Saint Domingue colonial society, whose members were eager consumers of popular science and devotees of new and interesting fads. Excited by the balloon flights of the Montgolfier brothers in 1783, residents flocked to witness similar launches in the colony. Awed by such wonders, the citizens of Saint Domingue were a receptive audience for news of scientific happenings.[9]

Colonists looked forward to the arrival of Count Antoine-Hyacinthe-Anne de Chastenet de Puységur, a mesmerist who had studied in Paris with the master himself after undergoing a successful treatment for asthma. His brother, the Marquis de Puységur, Armand-Marie-Jacques de Chastenet, was one of Mesmer's strongest provincial supporters. Assigned to the colony to complete a cartographic expedition in June 1784, Count Chastenet set up mesmerist tubs aboard ship, in the poorhouse of Cap-François, and in the magnetic society that he founded in Cap-François. He performed treatments there, and news of miraculous cures spread across the colony.[10]

The eagerness of Saint Domingue residents to embrace mesmerism demonstrates the precarious position that official European medicine held. One such enthusiastic proponent was long-time colonist, scientist, and intellectual Jean Trembley, who reported on the arrival of mesmerism in the colony to his friend and fellow naturalist and philosopher Charles Bonnet. Trembley, a planter known for his studies of plant and insect life in Saint Domingue, enjoyed discussing the latest scholarly issues with Charles Bonnet, who was best known for his study of aphids and his involvement in the preformationist and epigenist debate. In letters that rank Trembley as a first-class hypochondriac, he revealed to Bonnet the activities of Count Chastenet and the reaction the mesmerist received in Saint Domingue. Amidst talk of his latest headache and body pain, Trembley recounted Chastenet's arrival in the colony. He noted that Chastenet set up *baquets*, applied mesmerist treatments, and healed many men and women. Trembley described "A crippled man carried from the plain of the Cap on a stretcher, walked freely afterward." Trembley verified that mesmerism had roused the colony, which was abuzz with talk of the therapies. Trembley sympathized with the proponents of the technique, stating, "One cites many marvelous cures that cannot be attributed to the imagination."[11]

Madame Millet was another eyewitness to mesmerism in Saint Domingue. In fact, she revealed that she was a participant: "A magnetizer has been in the colony for a while now, and, following Mesmer's enlightened ideas, he causes in us effects that one feels without understanding them. We faint, we suffocate, we enter into truly dangerous frenzies that cause onlookers to worry." Madame Millet not only reported a loss of self-control to the sister with whom she corresponded, but also gave details of the sexual permissiveness that magnetism produced, a factor that had led to the therapy's downfall in Paris. She gossiped, "A young lady, after having torn off nearly all her clothes, amorously attacked a young man on the scene. The two were so deeply intertwined that we despaired of detaching them, and she could be torn from his arms only after another dose of magnetism." The reversal of gender norms (a young female assaulting a male) upset the assembled group, and, in order to combat the sexual confusion, they zapped the dangerous woman with a jolt of magnetism. With a twinge of reluctance and a show of proper female behavior, Millet conceded, "You'll admit that such are ominous effects to which women should sooner not expose themselves." Millet based her conclusion less on the fact that women should not enjoy the delirious feelings the therapies produced than on the risk of "a maltreated lover using it to his advantage."[12]

Despite positive response from some of Saint Domingue's leading citizens, practitioners of regular medicine, especially Charles Arthaud, bitterly attacked mesmerism as soon as it made its appearance in Saint Domingue. Arthaud was not one to shy away from an intellectual debate, especially when it concerned the official practice of medicine in the colony. Arthaud styled himself the colony's spokesmen on medical issues. Arthaud reviled mesmerist practice and, in 1784, joined forces with botanist Alexandre Dubourg and surgeon J. Cosme D'Angerville to form an ad hoc colonial investigatory committee. Their conclusion echoed the report made by the royal commission in France: Mesmerism was a dangerous hoax. Arthaud, Dubourg, and D'Angerville welcomed the opportunity to render their judgment. Even though leading physicians and surgeons swiftly rejected magnetism, they profited professionally from its existence. Their participation in the colonial mesmerist controversy demonstrated their understanding of current events and their adherence to metropolitan rhetoric. The debate over the merits of mesmerism increased their visibility within the colony and affirmed their tendency to speak for their fellow colonists. As a result of what they perceived as a victory over mesmerism, they established the colonial scientific and medical society known as the *Cercle des Philadelphes,* an institution that dominated colonial medicine and science for the remainder of France's rule in Saint Domingue.[13] Despite the commission's firm repudiation of mesmerist activity, mesmerism continued, making its way onto the plantations and into the slaveholding areas of the colony. The ad hoc committee's conclusion was correct—it was definitely dangerous. They had been concerned mainly with the hazards it presented to French and white Creole men and women; the colonists were soon to realize the perils mesmerism might produce when employed by enslaved men and women interested in promoting and giving voice to an ideology of rebellion and freedom.

"Nocturnal and Numerous Assemblies": *Mesmerism on the Plantations and among the Slaves*

Eager to maximize profits and to cut medical costs, some slaveholders and slave traders constructed mesmerist tubs and administered therapy on their slaves. The use of mesmerism by slaveowners is, of course, not surprising when one considers the tendency on the part of slaveholders to practice domestic medicine through the study of medical handbooks, via the application of patent remedies, and by way of advice given by plantation surgeons. Their gravitation toward mesmerism is simply another instance of them seeking to control the practice of medicine on the plantations. One plantation manager wrote to his boss that mesmerist techniques would benefit slaves "who have the greatest need for them."[14] Success stories, like the 1785 report of a female slave who won a decade-long battle with paralysis after undergoing mesmerist treatment, likely intensified a planter's willingness to try the technique.[15] Similarly, a crafty slave buyer mesmerized a cargo of slaves that he purchased at an exceedingly low price. After the treatment, he reported them to be in outstanding health and rented them out for fees normally reserved for only the best slaves.[16]

By 1786 mesmerism infiltrated the slave community. One region galvanized by slave magnetism was Marmelade, an area new to agricultural and economic development. Over 150 coffee plantations dotted the mountainous yet fertile soil of Marmelade; farms devoted to food production also existed. Seven thousand slaves, 500 whites, and 150 *affranchis* resided in the region. The majority of slaves were African, specifically Congolese, not Creole. A militia of 220 armed men was responsible for law and order, and a series of roads and a postal system kept Marmelade in contact with Cap-François.[17]

Official documents described the presence of mesmerism in the Marmelade region by noting

> a plantation manager, who had charge of eighty to one hundred slaves, called for a slave at two o'clock in the morning, and not gaining a response, must have been surprised and at the same time frightened to find out that the plantation was absolutely deserted.
> Another manager, no less alarmed when excited by a thud, hurried to the houses of the slaves, and found an assembly of five to six times as many slaves as actually lived on the plantation.[18]

The court records played on the fears of white slaveholders and their employees in a number of ways and demonstrated the dangerous quality of mesmerism. First, the plantation manager indicated that the command he gave was not heeded; the slave for whom he called was not available. Second, the manager revealed the plantation was deserted; enslaved men and women left without permission, an illegal act. If only one plantation manager had encountered this problem, the whites might not have had much to fear, but the court report continues with testimony given by another employee who worked on another plantation. While the first man was astonished by silence and desertion, the second endured loud noise and the presence of a large crowd of unknown slaves in a region with a large population of African slaves and a small number of white residents.

As a result of their interest in mesmerism, slaves engaged in simple acts of rebellion—they disregarded authority, disappeared without permission, and participated in an unauthorized assembly. These minor deeds of defiance grew more dangerous.

Seeking to put an end to the practice, in May 1786, the *Conseil Supérieur* of Cap-François prohibited

> the practice of magnetism to all those of African descent, free or not . . . an instrument that physics itself handles with precaution, which is easy to abuse and is apt for the tricks of jugglers who are common among the blacks and respected by them . . . taken over by them under the name of Bila . . . which might indicate just how far initiates or convulsionaries, of the class of Macandals, might take their mad fanaticism.[19]

The conclusions reached by the colonial ad hoc committee on mesmerism influenced the formulation of this law. The members of the court said that physicians recognized the dangers of mesmerism. They also identified the practice as being adopted by a group of slaves known as "jugglers," a term that referred to practitioners of spiritual medicine. The decree by the *Conseil* revealed the fear of macandalism that still existed nearly thirty years after the execution of its namesake and supports the contention that Makandal remained a symbol of rebellion and freedom years after his death, throughout the Haitian Revolution, and centuries afterward.

At least four slaves led the assemblies that distressed the residents of Marmelade. A biracial magnetist, Jérôme, and his black associate, Télémaque, both of whom were slaves belonging to Sieur Bellier, along with slaves Jean and Julien, were responsible for nighttime assemblies. The sources that reveal the story of the enslaved mesmerists are few, yet rich and varied. They include Moreau de Saint-Méry's report in *Description Topographique,* an account given by Gressier de la Jalousière (a resident of Marmelade), and the indictment presented to the *Conseil Supérieur du Cap.* The first and second mention only Jérôme and Télémaque, while the last accuses all four enslaved men. The amount of testimony tendered against them identifies Jérôme and Télémaque as the major actors in the mesmerist drama.[20]

Both whites and slaves, many of whom were house slaves and thus high-ranking slaves, testified against the slave magnetizers.[21] The fact that slaves took the stand against their fellow slaves is important for a number of reasons. Their testimony allows us to hear the voice of the enslaved, a sound and source that historians rarely get the privilege of experiencing. In addition, the information provided by enslaved men shows that the slave community was divided into factions, most especially because of the differences that existed between house slaves and field slaves. Finally, slave testimony indicates that slaves were not afraid to intimidate other slaves by providing testimony or by employing violence against slaves considered disloyal to a cause.

The unlawful meeting of slaves in an area populated overwhelmingly by slaves of African descent troubled those who kept records of the Marmelade magnetism controversy. They indicate that the nighttime gatherings were numerous and well attended. Gressier de la Jalousière revealed that there were "assemblies of slaves in the banana groves and in other hidden places and always at night."[22] Moreau de Saint-Méry described them as "secluded" and "immense."[23] The testimony by witnesses who appeared before the Superior Court of Cap-François echoed the descriptions given by Gressier de la Jalousière and Moreau de Saint-Méry. They used phrases like "nocturnal and numerous assemblies," and "considerable assembly." Some eyewitnesses identified specific participants. An enslaved man named Scipion stated that "he knew Jean perfectly well for having seen him come often on the plantation of his master in the company of the mulatto Jérôme with whom he held the assemblies." Another slave, Philippe, verified Scipion's statement by noting that he often saw Jean at Jérôme's house and at the assemblies. Perhaps the most damning accusation was made by Sieur Desplas, who talked of "numerous assemblies" held at a neighboring plantation and one so tumultuous that he was forced to go there in order to scatter those assembled. Desplas's account is the most frightening to the court because the assemblies were so out of control that Desplas traveled to a nearby landholding to chase the slaves away.[24] All the records bear witness to the secrecy that surrounded the gatherings—they took place at night and in the hidden recesses of the plantations.

The clandestine nature of the assemblies alarmed the white and black residents of Marmelade; they were also concerned about the movement of slaves between plantations. Scipion and Philippe stated that Jean was seen at Jérôme's house and at the plantation on which Jérôme worked. Sieur Henry Estève and his slave Jasmine reported that Jean not only traveled away from his home to attend these meetings but sent out his underlings to search for plants, including the branches of the avocado tree, to be used during rituals.[25] Various laws prohibited slaves from assembling or traveling away from their plantations.[26] The spread of the therapies also shocked eyewitnesses. A large number of plantations seemed to be affected not only in Marmelade but elsewhere.

The mysterious ceremonies that took place at the midnight gatherings puzzled eyewitnesses even more than the size of the meetings and the travel undertaken by the slaves. Sieur Jacquin recounted, "He saw . . . the slave Jean in the middle of a considerable assembly, the said slave on his knees in front of a table covered by a rug and lit by two candles, raising a fetish."[27] The plantation manager made sure to mention the two machetes, crossed and on the ground in front of Jean. An enslaved man named Dimanche described a ritual in which "the participants held the leaves of the raspberry bush, the avocado tree, and the orange tree in their hands, knelt, and drank tafia mixed with spices." The participants then fell and Jean lifted them up by striking them with the machete.[28]

The assemblies and the ceremonies that took place at them surely baffled those who witnessed them and those who heard reports of them. Even more of a problem was evidence that slave leaders were gaining associates. These initiates, whom Moreau de Saint-Méry described as "feeble, superstitious men," not only collected herbs but also participated in the same activities and embraced the same ideals as their leaders.[29] Representatives of the court assumed a paternalistic tone on behalf of the "imbecilic and credulous multitude, seduced and fooled by skillful jugglers, cunning charlatans."[30] By describing the slaves who attended the ceremonies as weak, the white commentators sought to assume power over them in order to protect them from the magnetizers.

The mesmerists and their initiates sold sacred objects and performed rituals for pay. Jérôme distributed *maman-bila* (small limestone rocks) in sacks, *poto* (red and black berries of the acacia), and *mayombos* (batons filled with *maman-bila*). *Poto* cost a *gourde* (or five colonial *livres*), while *mayombos* cost four. If the *mayombos* were heavily decorated, they could sell for as much as 66 colonial *livres*.[31] One witness, Scipion, said "that Jean takes money . . . for performing ceremonies and for selling boxes to them."[32] Finally, the enslaved magnetists collected half the earnings gained by their assistants.[33] Sources do not reveal what the money was used to purchase. Perhaps it paid for the items—tafia, plants, and candles—used during the ceremonies. Weapons, including additional machetes, also may have been desired goods.

The ability to earn money and assume authority over their fellow slaves appealed to Jérôme, Télémaque, Jean, Julien, and their subordinates; the call for violent rebellion was even more exhilarating. Their message of freedom and liberty provoked only fear in the minds of whites and slaves who failed to pledge allegiance to these men. Sources bear witness to the rebellion preached by the mesmerists. They incited slaves to commit violence through the sale of talismans that they said would protect the wearer from attack by a slave who did not possess the magical charm.[34] Whites feared that the slaves would be led to conclude that the talismans might provide protection from violence perpetrated by white planters and soldiers. Machetes, agricultural utensils that could easily be used as weapons, figured prominently in the ceremonies. Eyewitnesses reported that these tools were not only essential items during ritual performances but also were carried by the slaves as types of arms. Sieur Lagarde, a surgeon, reported that during Jean's time as a runaway he chased the slave, who was armed with a machete and a stick.[35] The whites did not doubt that these items were being used as weapons; Moreau de Saint-Méry summarized the view of the colonists when he said that the mesmerists "all preached rebellion."[36]

The revolutionary message of the enslaved mesmerists disturbed colonial authorities, and they decided to bring the men to justice. According to the *Conseil Supérieur du Cap*, the magnetizers violated several laws, including the *Code Noir*, the royal decree of 30 December 1746, the colonial decree of 7 April 1758, and the colonial declaration of 16 May 1786. Taken together, these laws prohibited slaves from assembling and from making, selling, and distributing herbal remedies and talismans. The 1746 law demonstrated that the magnetizers were held to the same legal strictures that constrained enslaved healers from caring for their enslaved brethren and white clients. The magnetist controversy also renewed fears that emerged during Makandal's reign of terror. These fears are made plain by the court's willingness to apply the 1758 law, which stated, "Prohibited to free men of color and slaves to compose, sell, and distribute or buy talismans and *macandals*." Finally, the declaration of 1786 explicitly mentioned magnetism and forbade slaves and men and women of color from practicing it.[37]

Sources do not agree on the exact fate of the mesmerists. Moreau de Saint-Méry reported that Jérôme was sent to the galleys for life and Télémaque was subjected to the iron collar and exposed to the public. Since Moreau de Saint-Méry's information is secondhand, the records of the *Conseil Supérieur du Cap* are probably more accurate. They note the runaway status of both Jérôme and Télémaque. Because the men were fugitives, a punishment of hanging and strangulation was conducted in effigy. The ceremonial punishments were designed to serve as examples to other slaves who might think of opposing white rule. Jean unfortunately was imprisoned and endured the sentence handed down to Jérôme and Télémaque. The court decided "to condemn him to be hung and strangled until death follows." The lack of testimony against Julien preserved his life; the court decided that he assist at the other executions and then be sent back to his master. Julien's punishment was both psychological and physical. He participated in the cruelty inflicted on his comrade and likely received a severe beating once he was returned to his slaveowner.[38]

Why had the authorities reacted so harshly against the slave magnetizers? The repression of mesmerism among the slaves stemmed in part from the attitude of the scientific and medical elite of Saint Domingue toward mesmerism. They absolutely detested the practice of mesmerism and sought to put an end to it among the white residents of Saint Domingue. Yet Puységur, the French mesmerist who practiced in the poorhouses of Saint Domingue, was not subject to the violent physical punishment to which the enslaved men fell victim. To its detractors, mesmerism signified the dangerous breakdown of hierarchy and, what was most frightening, the potential destruction of Saint Domingue's slave society. The ceremonies to which the slaves flocked defied traditional notions of authority. The slaves violated many laws, not simply the one that prohibited them from practicing this newfangled therapy. They assembled, they ran away, they carried agricultural objects as weapons and were intent on using them, and they sold merchandise and pocketed the money for their own gain. The slaves also acted as healers, a role that was legally denied to them.

Was It Mesmerism?

The question remains: Were the slaves practicing mesmerism? We may never know. One key piece of information eludes us—an enslaved participant telling us that indeed the slaves were following the lead of their masters and practicing mesmerism. Historians rarely find so juicy a detail or so definitive an answer. The court records do describe the rituals as magnetism by using the phrase *"prétendu magnétisme,"* which one may translate as "so-called magnetism."[39] The tone that the court took seemed to be one of condescension toward the slave leaders. They believed that the ceremonies represented attempts by the slaves to participate in the mesmerist craze, but that these rituals fell short of the European original. The court also chose to describe the assemblies as mesmerist meetings in order to flex their legal muscle and utilize the declaration they had recently issued. The members of the legal body used a number of documents to find the men guilty, but the prohibition against mesmerism cannot be discounted or dismissed outright as the motive for bringing charges. The court believed that the slaves were practicing magnetism. At the very least, the charge of mesmerism made against the slaves by white authorities was a way for the court to bolster their case against wayward and dangerous slaves. The accusation of mesmerism also was an interesting story that colonial commentators like Moreau de Saint-Méry wrote about in order to prove that Saint Domingue was on the cutting edge of French science and medicine. Their ideas about and opposition to mesmerism matched the notions advanced by some of the greatest thinkers of the age.

The slaves themselves may have described the events in mesmerist terms. If slaves witnessed the excitement over magnetism and likened it to their own rites, they may have described their practices in the language of the slave masters. It was not uncommon for the residents of the colony, whether free, enslaved, black, white, or biracial, to be aware of the latest trends, to discuss them, and to participate in them. For example, fashion and the wearing of certain items of clothing cut across racial boundaries. White women emulated women of color, who took their cue from female slaves. Some historians argue that enslaved men and women in Saint Domingue heard talk of revolution while waiting on their masters at supper and that this unintentional communication of revolutionary ideology fomented rebellion and convinced the slaves to rise up and overthrow white rule. The same logic can be applied when considering mesmerism. White masters employed magnetism to deal with physical problems from which slaves suffered. Other European healing practices made their way into the Afro-Caribbean medical system created by slaves. Why should mesmerism have been so exceptional that it had not infiltrated the Creole culture constantly being refined and developed by the enslaved men and women of the island?

White witnesses reported that the slaves imitated mesmerist therapies but added unique elements to this European import. Those unique elements were likely vodou in origin. Anthropologist Alfred Métraux argued that vodou, like other practices, is subject to change. Métraux observed, "Vaudou . . . is a vital, living body of ideas and behaviors carried in time by its practitioners and responsive to the changing character of social life."[40] Scholars of vodou and its history repeatedly emphasize the ability of vodou to incorporate elements from disparate cultural systems.[41] Mesmerism definitely influenced vodou, as did the African origins of the slaves in Saint Domingue and the Caribbean environment into which these men and women had been thrust.

Evidence suggests that Jérôme, Télémaque, Jean, and Julien were vodou practitioners. Their ceremonies and symbolic objects are similar to certain aspects of vodou. The descriptions of vodou given by Moreau de Saint-Méry and other eighteenth-century authors correlate with the assemblies in which the enslaved mesmerists participated. The court proceedings related that, while holding various leaves, initiates drank tafia mixed with spices, fell to the ground, and were struck with a machete, which caused them to rise.[42] This ceremony is similar to Moreau de Saint-Méry's report of the *danse vaudou,* where new members remain possessed by a spirit until the priest strikes them with an object. The ritual, known as the putting-to-bed ceremony, continues today among vodou practitioners and initiates. Moreau de Saint-Méry spoke of another *danse* called *Danse à Don Petro,* which was reportedly created by a Spanish-born slave in Le Petit-Goave in 1786. During the dance, slaves consumed rum into which gunpowder was mixed. The dance became intense and was characterized by convulsive movements and chanting. The dance parallels Gressier de la Jalousière's report that Jérôme gave participants tafia mixed with gunpowder. The creation of this new dance was likely an outgrowth of the mesmerist craze that swept the colony in the mid-1780s and that touched the slave community in Marmelade.[43]

Just as Caribbean herbalism had been incorporated into the Afro-Caribbean pharmacopoeia developed by slaves, Caribbean religious elements also made their way into the formation of the Petro cult, the branch of vodou most intimately related to Haiti and its history. The magnetist controversy in Haiti occurred during the formation of this distinctive branch of vodou. The accused mesmerists Jérôme, Télémaque, Jean, and Julien appear to have been adherents and leaders of this cult. According to artist Maya Deren, the four leaders incorporated Caribbean religious symbolism into their ceremonies. As in the Petro cult, the table on which the leaders placed offerings was called a *bila.* This table is similar to the table on which the native people of Haiti, the Taino, worshipped their *zemis.* In addition, Deren asserted that that the *maman bila* sold by the practitioners may have derived from the name of the Carib snake deity, *mapoia* or *maboya.*[44] The pull of the Caribbean surroundings affected other aspects of vodou. In the northern part of Haiti the *lwa Zaka,* who wears the costume of the Haitian peasant farmer, is also called Mazaka, a name derived from *maza,* the Taino word for corn. Scholar Leslie G. Desmangles concluded, "The inclusion of the word [*zaka*] in Vodou mythology may have been the result of the maroon's contact with Indian culture in the interior of the island during the colonial period."[45] Desmangles also thinks that the *vèvès,* or the geometric drawings that symbolize the *lwas,* derive from Amerindian cultures.

Conclusion

Many residents of both Saint Domingue and France embraced magnetism because it offered them freedom from established medicine. Instead of therapies that depleted the body, mesmerism energized its adherents. Because the main opponents of mesmerism in Saint Domingue were official medical practitioners who had been appointed by the Crown, any action against their authority also was opposition against the state. The practice of mesmerism by slaves was a political act of revolution. In order to participate in magnetist treatments, slaves violated numerous restrictions—they ran away, they assembled, they traveled without permission, they practiced an illegal form of medicine, and they carried weapons. All these undertakings paid off in the slave rebellion of 1791. The mesmerist meetings in Marmelade were training grounds for revolution, and, thus, Anton Mesmer was onto something when he claimed that Haiti owed its independence to him.[46]

7 *The Transformative Power of the* Kaperlata

The blacks believe in magic and the empire of fetishes
follows them beyond the seas.
—Moreau de Saint-Méry, *Description Topographique*, 1797

In the eyes of French and Creole officials, the *kaperlata*s were
the most dangerous element of the medical underworld of eighteenth-
century Saint Domingue.[1] Using both natural and supernatural remedies,
they assumed great power among enslaved men and women and lower-
class whites and earned money through the sale of their herbal and spiritual cures. The *kaperlata* could be slave or free, man or woman. He or
she was not a recognized member of the plantation hierarchy and was,
in fact, greatly feared. Just like the fetishes they used, the identity of the
kaperlata transformed over time. Initially considered akin to sorcerers,
they practiced divination and distributed herbal remedies among slaves,
people of color, and lower-class whites. In the midst of revolution, colonial authorities deemed them dangerous influences with the potential
to destroy white society and grasp control of the island colony. Ultimately, the practices, power, and prestige associated with the *kaperlata*
became so great that the term was subsumed by practitioners of vodou
to identify a magical charm and the one who sold it.

Marie Kingué and the Kaperlatas

Marie Kingué was an enslaved woman and healer. Her patients trusted
in her ability to cure illnesses that were caused by evil spells. Witnesses

reported that she acted as a midwife and sold talismans. According to legal documents, she had assisted a pregnant woman who supposedly gave birth to a snake. The pregnant woman allegedly had been *Macandalisé*, or subjected to the mysterious power of the *macandalistes*. Documents also revealed that Marie "had the power to kill and raise from the dead, heal all sorts of maladies."[2]

Like other *kaperlata*s, Marie Kingué practiced divination and distributed herbal remedies among slaves, people of color, and lower-class whites. Divination is the practice of divining or foreseeing the future by established systems and processes, which can include the interpretation of a fixed body of information, the evaluation of objects shaken and thrown from a basket or bag, or an explanation based on spiritual possession of the diviner's body.[3] Kingué also sold talismans, one of the mainstays of the *kaperlata*'s healing repertoire. The men and women who purchased talismans believed that they protected the wearer from sickness brought on by magic. Moreau de Saint-Méry described the talismans "as small coarse figures of wood or stone" that "they call . . . garde-corps."[4] Finally she combined her work as a *kaperlata* with other healing techniques—she practiced midwifery and herbalism.[5]

Through divination and the manufacture and distribution of herbal remedies, charms, talismans, and potions, *kaperlata*s, like Marie Kingué, carried on an African healing tradition. Diviners occupied important places in Africa—he or she expressed, maintained, and validated the cultural truths of a society. Just as institutions, publications, and experimentation legitimized scientific and medical knowledge in eighteenth-century Europe, divination served as an epistemological foundation for many African cultural groups. Similarly, as Europeans under the influence of Linnaeus's taxonomic system rushed to classify natural objects, divination too provided a system of classification. Émile Durkheim and Marcel Mauss wrote, "The science of the diviners, therefore, does not form isolated groups of things, but binds these groups to each other. At the basis of a system of divination there is thus . . . a system of classification."[6]

As a result of the slave trade, various forms of African spiritual medicine made their way to Saint Domingue, leading to the creation of uniquely Afro-Caribbean forms of divination and spiritual healing that would eventually influence vodou practices. Moreau de Saint-Méry attributed the existence of *kaperlata*s in the colony to the fact that at least one-quarter of those sold into slavery in America had been accused of sorcery by their African neighbors. He also noted that this Afro-Caribbean form of supernatural medicine included "the odious art of poisoning."[7] Some *kaperlata*s did engage in individual and isolated instances of poi-

soning. More important, Moreau de Saint-Méry recognized the continu-
ance and transformation of African spiritual medical practices in Saint
Domingue that were comparable to the rise of *obeah,* or the use of spir-
itualism for evil purposes, and myalism, or medicine practiced to deal
with sorcery and witchcraft, in Jamaican slave society. From the legal
records that describe Kingué's case, one gets the sense that a similar division affected supernatural techniques in Saint Domingue. Kingué had
assisted an expectant mother who had been macandalized. Perhaps
Kingué's work as a *kaperlata* included methods designed to work against
the physical dangers posed by *macandalistes.* African slaves likely understood the difference between the two types of medical practitioners;
whites surely did not and identified both as sorcerers.[8]

The leaders of Saint Domingue society viewed Kingué as a threat because she developed a large following among the slaves and even among
members of the white community. Kingué also claimed to be free; the
transcript of her trial rejected her assertion stating that she was "in fact
a slave and a vagabond." She also repudiated part of her European name,
which was Marie Catherine, and chose instead to be called Marie Kingué.
She wanted to place herself outside the authority of the whites, and by
creating her own identity as a free woman with a different name, she assumed power over herself instead of being under the control of her master and whites like him. Finally, Kingué attributed to herself supernatural powers. Her political prowess, her audacity, and her ability to make
money through the sale of talismans angered the colonial elite. Legal
records describe her with very heated language, identifying her as "this
négresse, or rather this monster." As a result of the terror she inspired,
François Neufchateau, the *procureur* (attorney general) of Cap-François,
issued a warrant for her immediate arrest.[9]

Kingué's unfamiliar healing practices played a part in the pro-
nouncement made by whites that she and others like her practiced sorcery. European observers considered *kaperlata*s akin to sorcerers. There
were several reasons colonists labeled the techniques used by *kaperlata*s
as being on a par with witchcraft. For centuries, powerful members of
European society accused certain popular medical practitioners of working under the command of the devil. Specifically, impostors, or those who
pretended to possess a divine healing gift, and men and women who used
spells, incantation, and charms, not simply prayer, to heal were accused
of demonology and witchcraft and subjected to legal prosecution. These
traditional beliefs inspired the fears that whites had about the practices
of the *kaperlata*s.[10] Thus, the centuries-old crusade to eliminate popular
healers in France also was present in Saint Domingue.

White colonists, specifically professional medical practitioners and legal authorities, also disparaged the work of the *kaperlata*s because they simply misunderstood non-Western forms of medicine, which were unlike their own and which they associated with the work of European impostors and charm-sellers. Eighteenth-century medical science continued to look to the past for theories about disease, but the natural world and its objects, including plants and the human body, became the focus of scientific investigation and experimentation. The strange rituals of the *kaperlata*s seemed similar to religious ceremonies and traditions that were under attack by Enlightenment scholars as remnants of a bygone and irrational era. Proponents of the Enlightenment carried on the campaign to eliminate popular medical practitioners, but instead of viewing them as agents of the devil, they saw them as impostors who duped unknowing clients.[11]

Yet even the use by slaves of natural objects as medical remedies upset colonists. Whites opposed the practice of medicine by *kaperlata*s because of the anxieties they had about herbal medicine. The same remedies that offered relief from fevers, wounds, and scurvy might easily be turned against one's enemies. Thus, colonial authorities objected not only to the spiritual medicine practiced by *kaperlata*s but also to medical techniques that corresponded with the eighteenth century's search for answers from the natural world.

Stereotypes about Africans also shaped the apprehension that French men and women experienced over the work performed by *kaperlata*s. For centuries, the French had studied and drawn conclusions about Africans. The stereotype of the enslaved men and women as malicious, malevolent, and depraved creatures who used evil measures to achieve goals was a deep-seated European image of the African people.

First, scholars thought that men and women living in hot climates were subject to extreme physical sensitivity. The intense climate that African men and women experienced not only impelled them to engage in sexual promiscuity and other vices but sapped them of energy and made them easier for corrupt individuals to dominate. In addition, the nakedness of African men and women shocked European sensibilities, and this nudity quickly became associated with sexual wantonness and sin.[12] According to Europeans, the hypersexuality ascribed to Africans violated morality and made Africans subject to the whims of powerful figures. These notions led the French to conclude that African and Afro-Caribbean slaves naturally were attracted to the work of the *kaperlata*s, men and women who not only participated in what the French considered immoral activities, but also thrived on the power they had over their followers.

Second, the French highlighted the skin color of Africans in order to differentiate them from Europeans. This difference then became laden with cultural notions of right and wrong, moral and immoral behavior. The dark skin color of the African had long been associated in Europe with evil and evildoing. The ancient Greeks and Romans contrasted black, which signified death and dirt, with white, which indicated purity and life. The Church continued this tradition of associating blackness with evil; Christian scholars represented Satan himself in the guise of an African woman. As French contact with Africa and Africans increased in the seventeenth century, literary references to black as a symbol of evil reached a high point.[13] For Europeans, the practice of sorcery, or the work completed by *kaperlata*s, was itself defined by reference to color—it was a form of black magic.

The absence of Christianity among Africans supported the notion of the African as witch and sorcerer. Europeans concluded that unfamiliarity with Christianity or worse yet rejection of the faith were signs of victimization by and commerce with Satan. In the first half of the eighteenth century, French naval officer Dralsé de Grandpierre wrote that the African tendency to turn "ridiculous objects into gods . . . give us the right to consider them less as men than as animal."[14]

The accusation by whites that *kaperlata*s practiced sorcery and not an acceptable form of medicine also emerged from a place of fear. White colonists, especially colonial authorities and other members of the *grands blancs* class, worried about the dangerous influence that practitioners of spiritual medicine had on slaves, men and women of color, and lower-class whites. Moreau de Saint-Méry wrote, "A great number of blacks acquire absolute power over other slaves through sorcery and thus help themselves . . . to money, power, and possessions."[15] Records about Marie Kingué depicted the slaves who followed her in the same way that legal authorities portrayed the enslaved men and women who admired the magnetists. The devotees were duped by her, whom they "regarded . . . as a god." Maintaining their superior ability to think rationally, whites sought to gain control over the situation which they believed resulted from the naïveté of slaves. Despite the disparaging terms they used to describe Kingué's followers, whites did fear her power to amass a large following, which included men and women who, like Kingué, took leadership positions over fellow slaves. Official records clearly identify an enslaved man named Polidor as one of Kingué's lieutenants and the power he had over other slaves.[16]

The authority that *kaperlata*s had over men and women of color also frightened the colonists. Whites considered the *gens du couleur* as allies against the large population of enslaved men and women. In the minds of whites, the people of color were a buffer group that eased racial tensions between whites and blacks. Free interracial men served in the *maréchaussée* (militia), and one aim of this mounted police force was to pursue *maroons*. Whites supposed that a man of mixed race naturally excelled at this activity because he, like his black parent, possessed greater physical strength. Moreau de Saint-Méry claimed, "The Mulattos . . . who commonly pursue fugitive slaves . . . are superior to any other soldier. . . . [T]hey have the same advantages as the slave who uses his bare feet for ascending the steep rocks, or descending the sheer cliffs."[17] French colonists also employed men of color as paramilitary soldiers because the Europeans were well aware of and depended on the racial animosity that men of color had for slaves. According to whites, the tendency for people of color to seek the assistance of *kaperlata*s jeopardized the racial hierarchy that kept the French in charge. Outnumbered by slaves, whites feared the numerical strength that could be fielded by a combined force of enslaved people and men and women of color.

Colonial authorities also worried about lower-class whites associating with *kaperlata*s. The colony of Saint Domingue was divided not only racially but also economically. A minority of whites, the *grands blancs,* dominated the *petits blancs* politically, economically, socially, and culturally. Despite the benefits of race that *petits blancs* experienced, many lower-class whites struggled under the burdens of homelessness, economic instability, and the lack of a political voice. The spiritual and physical good fortune promised by the *kaperlata*s was an attractive offer. Outnumbered by African and Afro-Caribbean slaves, men and women of color, and whites of the lower class, the *grands blancs* were right to fear the power of the *kaperlata*s.

The Revolutionary Potential of the Kaperlatas

The revolution in Saint Domingue transformed life on many levels. The debate over political rights upset the colony's racial system as men of color demanded autonomy and slaves clamored for liberty. Colonists lost their livelihoods as plantations burned and slaves rebelled. The revolution not only affected the colonial economy, society, and political system, but also disturbed medicine. Because the Crown was under attack, the authority of the royally appointed medical practitioners was called into question. The disruption of the colony's racial hierarchy further weakened the ability of whites to exclude people of color and slaves from the practice of medicine. The identity of the *kaperlata* also transformed; in the midst of revolution, concerns over the *kaperlata*s came to include fears about the dangerous social and political influence posed by men of color who practiced medicine.

It is not surprising that the most vocal critic of the *kaperlata*s was Charles Arthaud. Writing during the French Revolution to the Committee of Public Health, the National Assembly, and the Colonial Assembly, Arthaud employed the figure of the *kaperlata* to discuss and argue against the participation of men of color in colonial medicine and in colonial society and politics.[18] Influenced by the dreams of the Medical Enlightenment, Arthaud saw the revolution as a unique opportunity to improve and perfect not only colonial medicine but colonial society. Arthaud and others like him believed that doctors would be the vanguard of a new, more perfect social order. He maintained that the colony of Saint Domingue could be improved through the efforts of its physicians.

Although he conceded that women of color and enslaved females might be allowed to continue their practice of midwifery, he wanted *kaperlata*s to have no place in his visionary colonial medical establishment. Drawing on earlier notions of the *kaperlata,* Arthaud described their techniques as "vulgar, superstitious, and often harmful."[19] He noted that the law of 1764 prohibited people of color and enslaved men and women from practicing medicine, but, as we know, both groups disregarded the law and acted as healers. He despised persons of color because of their unwillingness to obey colonial authorities, their use of different and, in his mind, dangerous therapies, and their economic success. He grudgingly acknowledged that they had a substantial clientele and that they employed remedies on themselves, their fellow people of color, and whites.

Arthaud wanted restrictions on the economic and social lives of people of color to continue. He believed that if they were allowed to practice medicine, they would damage the reputation of the medical profession. According to Arthaud, physicians demonstrated honor and delicacy when dealing with patients, and men of color lacked the ability to engage in such virtuous behavior. He also hinted at the importance of education to the medical profession; Arthaud's conclusion is apparent if not explicit—people of color did not possess the intellectual ability to pursue the studies necessary to become a physician. He also feared that *gens de couleur* would use their medical skills to seduce desperate families, who would then participate in conspiracies to improve the lot of men and women of color. Paranoid, Arthaud envisioned the ultimate outcome of allowing men of color to pursue medicine as a colony devoid of white authority and one where nonwhites "will be the sole proprietors of the Colony."[20]

Saint Domingue's Diseased Body Politic

Arthaud's identification of men of color as *kaperlata*s made use of popular imagery in the form of medical metaphors, which were being employed by writers to attack political opponents in both France and its
most important colony. At the end of the eighteenth century, political
theorists and social critics in France and elsewhere began to apply the
language of ill health to what they believed was wrong in their societies.
In other words, these scholars employed disease and medicine as metaphors. In France this descriptive and rhetorical device was used to attack
court life and to explain the French Revolution. Likewise, commentators used disease and medical metaphors to characterize the upheavals
in Saint Domingue that resulted, in large part, from the revolutionary
turmoil in the metropole. Inspired by a long tradition that compared the
state to the human body, eighteenth-century judges, political theorists,
and enslaved men and women described the colony of Saint Domingue
as being in the throes of a disease, compared political leaders with medical practitioners, and depicted military and political violence as wounds.
The colony's reputation for disease, its pathological system of slavery,
and its racially divided population created a unique vision of the Saint
Domingue body politic and the revolutionary fevers it endured.

The comparison of the political body to the human body is an ancient
element of political philosophy. This association, the organic analogy, has
been used from the time of the ancient Greeks to understand the organization and practice of power. In the fourth century B.C., Plato equated the
state with the body but expanded the analogy to include elements of sickness and health. In the *Republic,* he described the simple, rural state as
the healthy state, but one liable to fevers as a result of the public consumption of luxuries.[21] Greek folklorists like Aesop also built upon this
comparison by associating political unrest with bodily upset. In other
words, Greek thinkers saw political instability as a form of physical dis-
tress.[22]

The organic analogy continued to inform political notions in prein-
dustrial Europe. The medieval theory of "the king's two bodies" identified the monarch's body with the state. According to medieval scholars,
the monarch possessed two distinct bodies, a "natural body," which was
subject to illness and infirmity, and a "sacred body," which could not be
thwarted by bodily weakness but lived on in the "body politic" made up
of all the subjects of the realm.[23]

In the seventeenth century, English political theorist Thomas Hobbes
transformed the notion of the body politic through his promotion of so-

cial contract theory. Influenced by mechanistic conceptions of the natural world, Hobbes described the commonwealth as "an Artificial Man."[24] He argued that monarchy was not a natural form of government but originated through the desire of individuals to come together under one ruler for protection. Like Hobbes, eighteenth-century French philosopher Jean-Jacques Rousseau embraced social contract theory but saw sovereignty in the collective body of the people, not in the person of the king.[25] Both Hobbes and Rousseau noted the various "diseases" to which the body politic might fall subject.[26]

In the final years of the Ancien Régime, social critics began to use vocabularies of sickness and health in order to condemn the French court and its members for the troubles that existed in France. The most significant and eloquent deployment of medical language as a form of critique came from Louis-Sébastien Mercier, author of *Le Tableau de Paris* (*The Picture of Paris*). Mercier described the city of Paris as diseased, pathological, and a danger to the body politic. The inability of the city to ensure societal happiness resulted from its fetid environment and from the persons and organizations responsible for dirtying it. Such unhealthy individuals were the courtiers, who bestowed favors on select businessmen, speculators, and holders of monopolies. Mercier described such men and women as a "tapeworm" that eventually kills the being in which it lives. The remedy that Mercier prescribed in order to restore the health of the city and society in general was a large dose of freedom, or the right to think and trade freely.[27]

Disease and medical metaphors also did service during the Revolution. A medical lexicon informed the language of revolution because many medical practitioners were important and active members of the revolutionary middle class. Many saw the Revolution as a means to remedy the illnesses of the Ancien Régime. Likewise, words normally employed to characterize the ailing body or the body under medical care now came to be used to explain the revolutionary process. Examples of such terms include regime, constitution, degeneration, regeneration, convulsion, and purge. Titles like "charlatan," "empiric," and "mountebank" that originally disparaged fringe medical practitioners now designated individuals opposed to the perceived good of the nation.[28]

During the French Revolution, many French men and women expressed the dissatisfaction they felt for the French body politic by using medical metaphors. One of the most influential pamphleteers of the French Revolution, Abbé Emmanuel Sièyes, spoke of the crisis in France in surgical and medical terms. He described privilege as an unhealthy growth that depleted the energy of the nation. He claimed that only the most radical cure, amputation, would ensure the survival of France. By beheading King Louis XVI, revolutionaries had performed an operation designed to rid the political body of its diseased head.[29]

In Saint Domingue, the very real diseases that attacked the residents of the island, the actual practice of medicine, and the horrible wounds that resulted from the system of slavery informed the ways writers and residents of Saint Domingue employed the idea of the body politic. Just as physicians believed that the island produced unique physical ailments in the colonists and the colonized, the description of the Saint Domingue body politic included maladies like racism that were peculiar to the colony. Legal authorities also portrayed the practice of magnetism by slaves as a type of disease that needed to be expelled from the Saint Domingue body politic. Court records describe the rise of mesmerism as "a new disorder, rapid in its progress, which in a short amount of time will be one of those terrible sicknesses that is dangerous to attack and impossible to cure." They identified the source of infection as magnetist assemblies stating that "it is there that the Contagion is able to spread."[30]

The years of brutality and disease that slaves endured convinced them that the Saint Domingue body politic needed to be physically ripped apart. In the eyes of the slaves, disease was not an enemy, but an ally. As a result, African and Afro-Caribbean slaves employed disease to resist the power held by the colonial overseers and planters through reproductive resistance, suicide, self-mutilation, feigned illness, and poisoning.

Suicide was the most radical form of resistance that slaves practiced in order to physically escape the horrors of slavery. Many slaves took their own lives during the Middle Passage to free themselves from the physical and psychological tortures they experienced trapped below deck. An especially high rate of suicide was observed among the Ibo people of West Africa. The "Coromantine" slaves (the Akan-speaking residents of modern Ghana) also engaged in suicide as a form of mass resistance aboard ship and once they reached their Caribbean destination. Slaves succeeded in taking their own lives by refusing to eat or drink, by throwing themselves overboard, and by hanging themselves. Descourtilz reported that suicide was common in Saint Domingue because "the blacks of certain African nations are strongly persuaded that by killing themselves they will return without fail to the country where they were born."[31] Slaves who took their own lives put faith in a West African religious belief that saw suicide as a means of gaining freedom, not as an act of desperation. Other enslaved men and women looked to suicide as a way to seek revenge on the living. This type of self-destruction, particular to animist religion, had as its goals the return of the deceased's spirit and the torture of those persons who had offended the dead and pushed him or her to the act of suicide.[32]

Self-mutilation was another form of biological resistance that took place in Saint Domingue. Slaves resorted to damaging their bodies to escape the backbreaking labor they were forced to complete. The tale of Jean-Baptiste exemplifies this type of resistance. According to an account published by Moreau de Saint-Méry, Jean-Baptiste detested working his master's fields. He decided that he could avoid this labor by cutting off his right arm. Moreau reported that the enslaved man succeeded only on the fourth attempt.[33]

Accidental mutilation, like that experienced by Makandal, also fueled revenge against one's master and whites in general. Slaves who fed sugar into rollers and who utilized sharp farming utensils could be severely injured. As a result, their work as field laborers was effectively terminated, and they moved into positions that gave them greater time alone or more contact with members of the white family and their belongings. Slaves took this time and opportunity to resist the power of their master through acts of resistance like poisoning.

Forms of resistance less drastic than suicide and self-mutilation also existed. Slaves feigned illness to avoid work, to gain much-needed rest by being confined to the slave quarters or by being housed in the plantation hospital, and to frustrate the economic goals of their masters. Planters and their employers also accused enslaved women of faking "female complaints" and using nursing to free themselves from labor in the fields.[34]

Slaves employed disease, or bodily harm, as a form of resistance because they understood that the most valuable weapons they had at their disposal were their own bodies and the bodies of other slaves. Slaves harmed themselves to gain freedom from servitude or to lessen the work expected of them. Slaves who feigned illness did so in order to gain rest and to frustrate the economic goals of their masters by denying them labor. Enslaved mothers chose to abort their babies and practiced infanticide in order to refuse their masters more laborers. Slaves like Makandal who engaged in poisoning, likewise, participated in biological terrorism. By striking out at the enslaved body, these men and women also lashed out at the Saint Domingue body politic, a political, economic, and social entity based upon physical differences between the three main groups of inhabitants—whites, men and women of color, and slaves.

Whites saw enslaved healers as the main participants in this attack on the Saint Domingue body politic. As a result, the distinctive medical practitioners and practices at work in the colony informed the characterizations of revolutionary political leaders, both free and enslaved. British historian, Jamaican planter, and proslavery parliamentarian Bryan Edwards, for instance, feared the rise of revolutionaries, whom he denigrated as "mountebanks," a label usually reserved for unlicensed and unscrupulous medical practitioners.[35] Employing the medical rhetoric of the Enlightenment, observers attributed the revolution that swept away French rule to the work of "charlatans" and "pestilent reformers," whom they held responsible for the "wounds . . . green and bleeding" that destroyed Saint Domingue.[36] Similarly, Arthaud's decision to describe people of color who practiced medicine as *kaperlata*s played to the fears and prejudices of his audience. To Europeans, *kaperlata*s were akin to sorcerers—dangerous practitioners of black magic and possible poisoners. In addition, drawing on widespread stereotypes about people of color, Arthaud described them as seductive and conspiratorial. According to white colonists, people of color, in particular biracial women, were bewitching creatures whose charms resulted in the impoverishment of white men and their families. If people of color served as physicians to white families, they would use their natural charms, not sound learning, to infiltrate, dominate, and ultimately destroy these domestic units, white power, and the Saint Domingue body politic. In Arthaud's eyes, and in the minds of other witnesses, medicine was power.

The Continuing Influence of the Kaperlata on Vodou and Haiti's History

Like other enslaved healers, *kaperlata*s contributed to the formation of a new cultural system through the influence that they had on vodou. As we have seen, enslaved healers like Makandal, the *macandalistes,* and the magnetizers participated in and affected the development of vodou rituals. There is also evidence that *kaperlata*s like Marie Kingué may have been involved in what would eventually be described as vodou. She was likely a practitioner of vodou, perhaps even a Vodou Queen. Kingué's ability to raise men and women from the dead may refer to the use of drugs that produce a zombielike state and the "resurrection" of an individual from this physical state.[37] In addition, testimony revealed that she assisted a pregnant woman who gave birth to a snake. The serpent was an important symbol in vodou ritual. According to Moreau de Saint-Méry, followers believe that "Vaudoux signifies a very powerful and supernatural being on which depend all the events that pass on earth. This creature is a nonvenomous serpent, or a species of snake, and it is under its patronage that all assemble together to profess the same doctrine."[38]

Not only did *kaperlata*s like Marie Kingué participate and shape vodou, but their very identity and one of their major therapeutic techniques became part of vodou vocabulary. The vodou terms *caprelata* and *caprelateur* refer to a "magic charm" and "magician who makes *caprelata*" respectively. Thus, one of the major medical techniques provided by enslaved practitioners of medicine, the creation and distribution of amulets, became a significant part of the vodou ritual. Just as slaves wore talismans to protect the wearer from physical violence perpetrated by both human and supernatural beings, Haitians still wear them as a defense against physical and spiritual dangers.

Conclusion: The Influence of the Enslaved Healers— Yesterday, Today, and Tomorrow

The enslaved healers of eighteenth-century Saint Domingue continue to inspire men and women in Haiti. The most telling example of their power is an elderly man by the name of Frédéric Géromi, who is also known as Véxémoi. Like the enslaved healers, Géromi has emerged as a leader in the small village of Baudin through a process of cultural retention, assimilation, and creation and has profited economically from his healing practices. The example set by him and by the enslaved healers teaches that marginalized medical practitioners throughout the world hold the key to transforming the communities in which they live.

The enslaved healers offered a great many services to their clients in several locations; Géromi does likewise. *Hospitalières* worked in plantation hospitals and yaws huts, where they mended broken bodies and distributed medicines. Midwives cared for pregnant, laboring, and nursing mothers and their children in the homes of their patients and in lying-in hospitals. *Infirmières* completed their tasks in the fields and in plantation hospitals. They assisted *hospitalières* but also provided pediatric and podiatric care to the third work gang, which was made up of young slaves. Working outside the institutional parameters of the plantation, herbalists dispensed a variety of drugs that could be used to treat wounds, fevers, and scurvy. Like the *kaperlata*s, they combined spiritual and herbal healing. *Gardiens de bêtes* treated creatures in plantation animal hospitals and in the fields, where they restored wounded and ailing animals and where they provided both routine and emergency care. Their associates, the *pacotilleurs*, ministered to human and nonhuman animals using the plants that thrived in the colony. As country doctor, herbalist, and midwife, Monsieur Géromi cares for his neighbors in multiple ways. As a country doctor, he ministers to the medical needs of his neighbors. As an herbalist, he concocts remedies that help to ease stomach pains and creates medicines that aid in the healing of fractured bones. As a midwife, he tends to pregnant women and their infants.

The labor undertaken by enslaved healers allowed them to retain elements of African healing traditions, to appropriate Western and Caribbean medical techniques, and to contribute to an Afro-Caribbean health care system. Their work as enslaved healers echoed African social roles. *Hospitalières* utilized African inoculation procedures and employed African methods to treat worm infestation. Midwives applied African birthing and postnatal care procedures. Herbalists offered plant remedies that were more familiar to African and Creole slaves than the medicines distributed by the master and his white employees. *Kaperlatas* looked to African divination practices to tend to their clients. *Gardiens de bêtes* relied on traditional African veterinary knowledge. Enslaved healers did absorb elements of native Caribbean and Western therapeutics. Enslaved women who tended to slaves housed in the plantation hospital became familiar with remedies compatible with Western humoral medicine. Magnetizers used the language of mesmerism to promote their healing strategies. Veterinary artists received training from masters who were veterinary specialists themselves. In the final analysis, enslaved healers employed therapies that combined African, European, and Caribbean medicine. Similarly, Géromi employs both Afro-Caribbean and Western medical therapies and techniques. Like his ancestors, he grows the plants that he uses as remedies in his garden. He follows the directives of government officials who publish pamphlets on the best ways to render prenatal and postnatal care. He assists at a local dispensary staffed every few months by Western medical aid workers and accepts the tools and medicines they give him at the end of their brief stays.

Géromi's training also resembles the preparation received by the medical men and women of the eighteenth century, who learned their craft from more experienced and older practitioners. His first teacher was his grandmother, who was, like him, a village healer. It was perhaps from her that Géromi learned that *mal-de-mère* could be used to treat pregnant women, an application of the herb that enslaved healers, likewise, knew and employed. Géromi combined his grandmother's lessons with study at a seminary, where he received official certification to provide medical care and to serve as a midwife. He proudly displays his license to practice to Western observers.

Slaves who practiced the healing arts profited politically and economically from their practices. Healers on the plantation, including midwives and hospital administrators, occupied the most powerful positions that female slaves held within the plantation hierarchy. They benefited from extra food, clothing, and gifts. As a result of the important services they rendered, they were more likely than other female slaves to be granted both official and unofficial freedom. Slaves recognized herbalists, mesmerists, and *kaperlata*s as important political leaders. Healers translated their power into material gain. Marie Kingué, a midwife and *kaperlata*, sold talismans, and enslaved mesmerists collected money and goods in exchange for the rituals they performed and the items they sold. Like the enslaved healers, Géromi is a respected figure in Baudin. His centrality to his community is apparent in the location of his home, which is in the middle of the village across from the marketplace. His association with U.S. medical practitioners supplies him with money and much-needed medical supplies. Like enslaved healers who gained freedom for themselves and their children through the services and goods they sold, Géromi's actions and visibility have affected the life of his daughter, who hopes to pursue medical studies through the sponsorship of U.S. patrons.

White colonists eyed enslaved healers suspiciously because of their ability to resist the slave system. Colonial authorities passed laws that prohibited or limited the ability of healers to care for fellow slaves and white residents. Plantation managers and surgeons held positions of authority over female practitioners and were unafraid of disciplining and punishing them when the *hospitalières,* midwives, and *infirmières* were accused of or found guilty of occupational sabotage. Fearing poisoning undertaken by herbalists and veterinary artists, whites subjected these healers to torture by forcing them to ingest strange and unknown substances. Court proceedings attempted to curb the power of the mesmerists and *kaperlata*s. Géromi too is treated harshly by some Western relief workers, who regard him as a danger to the men, women, and children whom he treats. Although he utilizes modern medical techniques, his use of traditional remedies appears to some to be a throwback to earlier, more dangerous times. Géromi's marginality also emerges when he deals with the Haitian religious sisters who operate the village medical clinic. Thus, Géromi struggles with two influential forces within Haiti and within his small village: the Roman Catholic Church and the U.S. relief workers.

The enslaved healers were medical revolutionaries in two important ways. First, they contributed to the creation of an Afro-Caribbean medical system, aspects of which were incorporated into the Western medical tradition. Second, they participated in acts of rebellion that laid the foundation for the Haitian Revolution. Their fellow slaves and future revolutionaries were inspired by their daring actions and joined them in their fight against slavery and in the eventual expulsion of the French from Haiti. Their story draws attention to the power of medical practitioners to effect political, economic, and social change. The history of medical revolutionaries demonstrates that marginalized medical practitioners can transform the communities in which they live. Ethnomedical researchers argue that traditional medicine, both human and nonhuman, will have a greater effect on improving the well-being of local communities than the imposition of foreign medical practices and therapies. The majority of biomedical and pharmacological research does not concern the major health problems from which people in developing countries suffer. Like the medical therapies of the enslaved healers, the medical techniques of traditional practitioners incorporate many forms or traditions of medicine that diverge radically from Western biomedicine.[1] If the revolutionary legacy of the enslaved healers is to continue to bear fruit in Haiti and in other areas of the globe, it will be through the work of men and women like Frédéric Géromi.

NOTES

Introduction

1. Sheridan, *Doctors and Slaves.*
2. Leti, *Santé et Société.*
3. Savitt, *Medicine and Slavery;* Bankole, *Slavery and Medicine.*
4. Pluchon, *Vaudou Sorciers.*
5. Debien, *Plantations;* Debien, *Esclaves.*
6. McClellan, *Colonialism and Science.*
7. McClellan and Regourd, "Colonial Machine."
8. Moitt, *Women and Slavery,* 62.
9. Arnold, "Tropical Medicine before Manson," Introduction to *Warm Climates and Western Medicine.*
10. For examples of resistance studies in the United States and the Caribbean, see Beckles, *Natural Rebels;* Hall, *Social Control;* Moitt, *Women and Slavery;* J. Morgan, *Laboring Women;* P. Morgan, *Slave Counterpoint;* Mullin, *Africa in America.*
11. Philip Morgan argues that formation of culture by American slaves simultaneously resisted and supported slavery (*Slave Counterpoint,* xxii).
12. Beckles, *Natural Rebels;* Moitt, *Women and Slavery;* and J. Morgan, *Laboring Women.*
13. Desmangles, *Faces of the Gods;* Fick, *Making of Haiti.*
14. Geggus, *Haitian Revolutionary Studies.*
15. Scott, *Domination,* 192.
16. Beckles, *Natural Rebels;* Bush, *Slave Women;* and Moitt, *Women and Slavery.*

Chapter 1: Saint Domingue

1. Lewis, *Main Currents in Caribbean Thought;* Stannard, *American Holocaust.*
2. Moreau de Saint-Méry, *Description Topographique.*
3. James, *Black Jacobins.*
4. Moreau de Saint-Méry, *Description Topographique.*
5. McClellan, *Colonialism and Science.*
6. Ducoeurjoly, *Manuel des Habitans;* Raynal, *Essai.*
7. For a discussion of the commercial economy of Saint Domingue in the eighteenth century, see James, *Black Jacobins;* Pluchon, *Toussaint Louverture;* and Stein, *French Sugar.*
8. Laborie, *Coffee Planter.* For secondary source analyses, see J. Brown, *History*

and Present Condition; Fick, *Making of Haiti;* James, *Black Jacobins,* 46; and McClellan, *Colonialism and Science.*

9. Laborie, *Coffee Planter.*

10. Raynal, *Essai.*

11. Moreau de Saint-Méry, *Description Topographique.*

12. Girod-Chantrans, *Voyage d'un Suisse.*

13. Moreau de Saint-Méry, *Description Topographique.* For a discussion of the political administration of Saint Domingue in the eighteenth century, see James, *Black Jacobins;* J. Brown, *History and Present Condition.*

14. Raynal, *Essai,* 14.

15. Laborie, *Coffee Planter,* Appendix, 97.

16. Raynal, *Essai.*

17. Moreau de Saint-Méry, *Description Topographique.* Thanks to Bill Hudon for informing me about the history of the Jesuits in the eighteenth century.

18. Métraux, *Voodoo.*

19. Ducoeurjoly, *Manuel des Habitans;* Laborie, *Coffee Planter.*

20. Moreau de Saint-Méry, *Description Topographique.*

21. Dayan, *Haiti;* Fick, *Making of Haiti;* James, *Black Jacobins;* and McClellan, *Colonialism and Science.*

22. Gautier, *Soeurs de Solitude.*

23. Moreau de Saint-Méry, *Description Topographique.*

24. James, *Black Jacobins.*

25. Moreau de Saint-Méry, *Description Topographique.*

26. Ducoeurjoly, *Manuel des Habitans.*

27. Laborie, *Coffee Planter.*

28. Ducoeurjoly, *Manuel des Habitans.*

29. James and Martin, *All Possible Worlds;* Nussbaum, *Torrid Zones.*

30. Dutertre, *Histoire Générale des Antilles,* 2: 64.

31. Labat, *Nouveau Voyage,* 1: 154. For biographical information about Labat, see McClellan, *Colonialism and Science.*

32. James and Martin, *All Possible Worlds;* Nussbaum, *Torrid Zones.*

33. Livingstone, *Geographical Tradition.*

34. Montesquieu, *Spirit of the Laws* (1758), 232.

35. Moreau de Saint-Méry, *Description Topographique,* 2: 516.

36. Bertin, *Des Moyens.*

37. Délorme, "Réflexions sur la Topographie," 2.

38. Poissonnier-Desperrières, *Traité sur les Maladies,* 325–26.

39. Pouppée-Desportes, *Histoire des Maladies,* 1: 195.

40. Poissonnier-Desperrières, *Traité des Fièvres,* 7, 10.

41. Bourgeois, *Voyages Intéressans,* 438.

42. Poissonnier-Desperrières, *Traité des Fièvres,* 91.

43. Pouppée-Desportes, *Histoire des Maladies,* 1: 40.

44. Bourgeois, *Voyages Intéressans;* Pouppée-Desportes, *Histoire des Maladies.*

45. Lafosse, *Avis aux Habitans,* 96.

46. For contemporary evidence of conditions aboard ship, see Duchemin de l'Étang, "Précautions à Prendre pour les Nègres," *Gazette de Médecine pour les Colonies* 3 (1 Dec. 1778), 13–15, CAOM, BMdSM, 87/MIOM/63. Text-fiche. Secondary source analyses include Alden and Miller, "Unwanted Cargoes," in Kipler, *African Exchange;* Debien, *Esclaves aux Antilles;* Kiple, *Caribbean Slave.*

47. Arthaud, *Observations sur les Lois*, 16–19, CAOM, 87/MIOM/41, BMdSM.

48. Moreau de Saint-Méry, *Description Topographique*, 1: 409–10.

49. Arthaud, *Observations sur les Lois*.

50. Kiple, *Caribbean Slave*.

51. Chevalier, *Lettres à M. de Jean*, 7.

52. Cauna, *Au Temps des Isles à Sucre*; Debien, *Esclaves aux Antilles*; Kiple, *Caribbean Slave*.

53. Debien, *Esclaves aux Antilles*; Girod-Chantrans, *Voyage d'un Suisse*.

54. Debien, *Esclaves aux Antilles*.

55. Girod-Chantrans, *Voyage d'un Suisse*, 142–43.

56. Debien, *Esclaves aux Antilles*.

57. LeCesne, *Procuration*, AN, T561, 1 May 1789. For secondary source analyses, see Debien, *Esclaves aux Antilles*; Kiple, *Caribbean Slave*.

58. Chandler and Read, *Introduction to Parasitology*.

59. Dazille, *Observations sur les Maladies des Nègres*, 107.

60. Dazille, *Observations sur les Maladies des Nègres*, 255.

61. Quoted in Currie, *Impartial Review*, 12. Also see Currie, *Description of the Malignant Infectious Fever*.

62. College of Physicians of Philadelphia, *Facts and Observations*.

63. Butler, "Some Contributions."

64. "Update on Acquired Immune Deficiency Syndrome."

65. Altema and Bright, "Letter to the Editor"; Boncy, et al., "Letter to the Editor"; Leonidas and Hyppolite, "Haiti and the Acquired Immunodeficiency"; Marx, "Acquired Immune Deficiency"; Moses and Moses, "Letter to the Editor."

66. Cineas, "Letter to Editor."

67. Greco, "Letter to the Editor," 516.

68. Barry, Mellors, and Bia, "Haiti and the AIDS Connection," 594.

69. Farmer, *AIDS and Accusation*.

Chapter 2: European Medicine in the Torrid Zone

1. Brockliss and Jones, *Medical World*.

2. Ibid.; Cunningham and French, *Medical Enlightenment*.

3. Brockliss and Jones, *Medical World*.

4. For secondary analyses of this transformation in slave health care, consult Debien, *Esclaves aux Antilles*; Gautier, *Soeurs de Solitude*.

5. Ramsey, *Professional and Popular Medicine*.

6. Arthaud, *Observations sur les Lois*.

7. For a brief discussion of humoral theory, see Ackerknecht, *A Short History of Medicine*.

8. McClellan, *Colonialism and Science*.

9. For a thorough analysis of the *Cercle des Philadelphes*, see ibid. *Tétanos* was the term applied to a condition that was most likely tetanus when applied to adults and either neonatal tetany or tetanus when applied to children.

10. Biographical information found in Blanche Maurel and Étienne Taillemite, "Index des Noms de Personnes," in Moreau de Saint-Méry, *Description Topographique*.

11. Brockliss and Jones, *Medical World*.

12. McClellan, *Colonialism and Science.*

13. For discussion of the responsibilities of the royal physicians, see Arthaud, *Observations sur les Lois.* Secondary analyses are Bordes, *Évolution des Sciences;* Léon, "Esquisse de l'Histoire"; McClellan, *Colonialism and Science;* Pluchon, *Histoire.*

14. Arthaud, *Observations sur les Lois.*

15. Ibid.

16. Ibid.; Charles Arthaud and J. Cosme D'Augerville, *Procès Verbal de Visite des Prisons Royales du Cap,* 22 Dec. 1786, AN, 27 AP 11, Dossier 3.

17. McClellan, *Colonialism and Science.*

18. Brockliss and Jones, *Medical World.*

19. Arthaud, *Observations sur les Lois,* 36.

20. Ibid.

21. Ibid.

22. McClellan, *Colonialism and Science;* Pluchon, *Histoire.*

23. Arthaud, *Observations sur les Lois,* 21–22.

24. Brockliss and Jones, *Medical World,* 485–487; McClellan, *Colonialism and Science,* 133; and Ramsey, *Professional and Popular Medicine in France,* 19, 50.

25. Brockliss and Jones, *Medical World;* Ramsey, *Professional and Popular Medicine.*

26. McClellan, *Colonialism and Science;* Pluchon, *Histoire.*

27. Pouppée-Desportes, *Histoire des Maladies.*

28. Gelfand, "Monarchical Profession"; McClellan, *Colonialism and Science.*

29. Baradat, *Certificate to Practice Surgery Presented to Pierre Didier,* 2 July 1774, Winterthur Manuscripts, Group 10, series A, DuPont Family Miscellany. Hagley.

30. Chevalier, *Lettres à M. de Jean;* Poissonnier-Desperrières, *Traité des Fièvres.*

31. Brockliss and Jones, *Medical World;* Porter, ed., *Cambridge Illustrated History of Medicine.*

32. Moreau de Saint-Méry, *Description Topographique.*

33. Brockliss and Jones, *Medical World,* 576.

34. Brockliss and Jones, *Medical World.*

35. McClellan, *Colonialism and Science.*

36. Pouppée-Desportes, *Histoire des Maladies,* 1: 50.

37. Chevalier, *Lettres à M. de Jean,* 6.

38. Arthaud, *Observations sur les Lois;* Moreau de Saint-Méry, *Lois et Constitutions.*

39. Moreau de Saint-Méry, *Lois et Constitutions.* The 1765 law reiterated the 1556 edict of King Henri II, which said that women must not hide their pregnancies, nor murder their children.

40. Moreau de Saint-Méry, *Lois et Constitutions.*

41. McClellan, *Colonialism and Science.*

42. Moreau de Saint-Méry, *Description Topographique; Gazette de Saint Domingue, Politique, Civile, Économique et Littéraire, et Affiches Américaines,* 15 Jan. 1791, CAOM, BMdSM, 87MIOM/72, 54.

43. Pluchon, *Histoire.*

44. Ibid.

45. Hilliard d'Auberteuil, *Considérations sur l'État,* 1: 138–39.

46. Moreau de Saint-Méry, *Description Topographique;* Pluchon, *Histoire.*

47. Moreau de Saint-Méry, *Description Topographique*; Bordes, *Évolution des Sciences.*
48. McClellan, *Colonialism and Science.*
49. Moreau de Saint-Méry, *Description Topographique,* 1: 489.
50. McClellan, *Colonialism and Science.*
51. Ibid.
52. Pouppée-Desportes, *Histoire des Maladies,* 1: 148
53. McClellan, *Colonialism and Science*; Pluchon, *Histoire des Médecins.*
54. Bourgeois, *Voyages Intéressans.*
55. McClellan, *Colonialism and Science.*

Chapter 3: Enslaved Healers on the Plantation

1. Geggus, "Slave and Free Colored Women"; Moitt, *Women and Slavery*; Moitt, "Slave Women and Resistance"; Moitt, "Women, Work, and Resistance"; J. Morgan, *Laboring Women.*
2. Geggus, "Slave and Free Colored Women"; Moitt, *Women and Slavery*; Moitt, "Slave Women and Resistance"; Moitt, "Women, Work, and Resistance"; J. Morgan, *Laboring Women.*
3. Moitt, *Women and Slavery.*
4. Geggus, "Slave and Free Colored Women," 262.
5. Evidence suggests that male *hospitaliers* managed hospitals without the supervision of a European medical practitioner and had the opportunity to receive specialized instruction. For more information, see Lafosse, *Avis aux Habitans*; *Gazette de Saint Domingue, Politique, Civile, Économique et Littéraire, et Affiches Américaines,* CAOM, BMdSM, 87MIOM/72, 1 Jan. 1791 (supp.), 17–18.
6. Debien, *Esclaves aux Antilles*; Moitt, *Women and Slavery.*
7. LeCesne, *Correspondance du Gérant,* AN, T561, 5 Aug. 1791; Debien, *Plantations et Esclaves.* For information on medical cookery, see Schiebinger, *Mind Has No Sex?*
8. Labat, *Nouveau Voyage,* 3: 431.
9. Laborie, *Coffee Planter,* 167.
10. Descourtilz, *Histoire des Désastres,* 103.
11. Dazille, *Observations sur le Tétanos.*
12. Dazille, *Observations sur les Maladies des Nègres,* 104–5.
13. McClellan, *Colonialism and Science.*
14. Pluchon, *Histoire.*
15. Lafosse, *Avis aux Habitans,* 129.
16. Debien, *Les Esclaves aux Antilles.*
17. Ducoeurjoly, *Manuel des Habitans.*
18. Lafosse, *Avis aux Habitans,* 129
19. Laborie, *Coffee Planter.*
20. Lafosse, *Avis aux Habitans,* 128.
21. Bordes, *Évolution des Sciences*; Debien, *Esclaves aux Antilles*; Debien *Plantations et Esclaves.*
22. Laborie, *Coffee Planter,* 94.
23. Ibid., 187.

24. Ducoeurjoly, *Manuel des Habitans;* Girod-Chantrans, *Voyage d'un Suisse.* For secondary source analysis, see Debien, *Esclaves aux Antilles.*

25. Labat, *Nouveau Voyage,* 2: 247. For biographical information about Labat, see McClellan, *Colonialism and Science.*

26. Bourgeois, *Voyages Intéressans,* 458–59.

27. McClellan, *Colonialism and Science.*

28. LeCesne, *Compte Général de Nègres,* AN, T561, Dec. 1789.

29. LeCesne, *Correspondance du Gérant,* AN, T561, 28 Jan. 1790.

30. LeCesne, *Correspondance du Gérant,* AN, T561, 10 May 1789, 28 Jan. 1790, 22 Oct. 1790.

31. LeCesne, *État d'Esclaves,* AN, T561, 1 Jan. 1791; LeCesne, *Procuration,* AN, T561, 1 May 1789.

32. Laborie, *Coffee Planter,* 167.

33. Ibid.

34. Ibid., 189.

35. *Affiches Américaines* 5, 3 Feb. 1768, 43; *Affiches Américaines* 40, 3 Oct. 1772 (suppl.), 479. Houghton.

36. Ducoeurjoly, *Manuel des Habitans,* 2: 45.

37. Chevalier, *Lettres à M. de Jean,* 47.

38. Bourgeois reported that this was common practice among the slaves. If the worm broke while exiting the skin, the part that remained in the body would cause a massive infection. Bourgeois, *Voyages Intéressans.*

39. Ducoeurjoly, *Manuel des Habitans.*

40. *Affiches Américaines* 3, 16 Jan. 1781, no page number. Houghton.

41. Laborie, *Coffee Planter.* For secondary source analyses, see Debien, *Esclaves aux Antilles;* Moitt, *Women and Slavery.*

42. McClellan, *Colonialism and Science.*

43. Provenchere, *Compte,* AN, T1113, Dossier 9, 1765; *État de l'Habitation de Madame de Chavanne,* AN, T210, Dossier 1, 4 May 1771; Petit de Villers, *Procuration,* AN, T561, 1 May 1789. Laborie's manual supports this assessment. He wrote, "Where the gang is rather numerous, the doctress must have an assistant, to learn the art under her direction, and to execute the works of drudgery." Laborie, *Coffee Planter,* 167.

44. LeCesne, *État d'Esclaves,* AN, T561, 1 Jan. 1791.

45. LeCesne, *Mouvemens,* AN, T561, June 1791.

46. Ducoeurjoly, *Manuel des Habitans.*

47. Bertin, *Des Moyens,* 103.

48. Ducoeurjoly, *Manuel des Habitans.*

49. Debien, *Esclaves aux Antilles.*

50. Dazille, *Observations sur les Maladies des Nègres;* Debien, *Esclaves aux Antilles;* Girod-Chantrans, *Voyage d'un Suisse.* Also see Kiple, *Caribbean Slave.*

51. LeCesne, *Correspondance du Gérant,* AN, T561, 30 Sept. 1790, 22 Oct. 1790, 14 Jan. 1791.

52. For information on the history of smallpox and efforts made to eradicate it, see Fenner et al., *Smallpox;* Hopkins, *Princes and Peasants.* For information on the history of smallpox in colonial settings, see Arnold, "Smallpox and Colonial Medicine," in *Imperial Medicine and Indigenous Societies,* ed. Arnold; Vaughan, "Slavery, Smallpox, and Revolution"; Winslow, *Destroying Angel.*

53. Dazille, *Observations sur les Maladies des Nègres*. For secondary source analyses, see Cauna, *Au Temps des Isles à Sucre;* Debien, *Esclaves aux Antilles.*
54. Debien, *Esclaves aux Antilles Françaises;* McClellan, *Colonialism and Science.*
55. Arthaud, *Mémoire sur l'Inoculation de la Petite Vérole* (Cap-François, 1774), CAOM, BMdSM, 87MIOM/63, 10. Text-fiche.
56. Moreau de Saint-Méry, *Description Topographique.* For secondary source analyses, see Debien, *Esclaves aux Antilles;* McClellan, *Colonialism and Science.*
57. Ducoeurjoly, *Manuel des Habitans.*
58. Genton, *Feuille d'Hôpital,* AN, Sous-série AB XIX 3355, May 1789; Genton, *H^{on} d'Agoult au Camp de Louis,* AN, Sous-série AB XIX 3355, 1 June 1789.
59. Planteaux, *Correspondance du Gérant,* AN, T561, 8 May 1789, 2 June 1789, 5 July 1789.
60. LeCesne, *Correspondance du Gérant,* AN, T561, 11 May 1790.
61. Moreau de Saint-Méry, *Description Topographique,* 60.
62. Kiple and King, *Another Dimension.*
63. Bush, *Slave Women;* Sheridan, *Doctors and Slaves.* Megan Vaughan ("Slavery, Smallpox, and Revolution") suggests that enslaved men and women, likewise, practiced inoculation in Ile de France (Mauritius).
64. Paul Erdman Isert, *Voyages en Guinée et dans les Iles Caraïbes en Amérique. Translaté de l'Allemand* (Paris, 1793), 221, CAOM, 87MIOM/15, BMdSM.
65. Arthaud, *Mémoire sur l'Inoculation,* 9.
66. Duchemin de l'Étang, "Inoculation," *Gazette de Médecine pour les Colonies* 5 (1 Jan. 1779): 30, CAOM, BMdSM, 87MIOM/63. Text-fiche.
67. Herbert, "Smallpox Inoculation in Africa." Also see Stewart, "Edge of Utility."
68. Ducoeurjoly, *Manuel des Habitans.* Also see Moitt, "Women, Work, and Resistance."
69. Debien, *Esclaves aux Antilles.*
70. Bush, *Slave Women;* Morrissey, *Slave Women.*
71. James, *Black Jacobins;* Lenman, "Colonial Wars."
72. Gautier, *Les Soeurs de Solitude.*
73. Quoted in Debien, *Plantations et Esclaves,* 128, 129. Also see Debien, *Esclaves aux Antilles.*
74. Girod-Chantrans, *Voyage d'un Suisse;* LeCesne, *État d'Esclaves,* AN, T561, 1 Jan. 1791. Also see Debien, *Esclaves aux Antilles;* Moitt, "In the Shadow"; Moitt, *Women and Slavery.*
75. Dazille, *Observations sur le Tétanos.*
76. Pouppée-Desportes, *Histoire des Maladies,* 3: 24. For a secondary source analysis of African women's knowledge of contraception, see Morgan, *Laboring Women.*
77. Morton, *Atlas.*
78. Chevalier, *Lettres à M. de Jean;* Dazille, *Observations sur les Maladies des Nègres,* 54; Dazille, *Observations sur le Tétanos;* Gardane, *Maladies des Créoles.*
79. Bush, *Slave Women.*
80. Girod-Chantrans, *Voyage d'un Suisse,* 137. For secondary source analysis, see Bush, *Slave Women.*
81. Moitt, *Women and Slavery;* Moitt, "Slave Women and Resistance."

82. Brockliss and Jones, *Medical World*; Schiebinger, *Mind Has No Sex?*
83. Dazille, *Observations sur le Tétanos*. The work that Dazille wrote was *Observations sur la Santé des Femmes Enceintes entre les Tropiques; . . .*, which he included in *Observations sur le Tétanos*.
84. Chevalier, *Lettres à M. de Jean*, 37.
85. Ducoeurjoly, *Manuel des Habitans*.
86. Mintz, "Slave Life," discusses how slaves simultaneously practiced accommodation and resistance to slavery.
87. Historian Geneviève Leti (*Santé et Société*) notes that in Martinique the *hospitalière* embodied the interpenetration of African and Western medicine. The same can be said for the *hospitalières* of Saint Domingue.
88. McClellan, *Colonialism and Science*; Morrissey, *Slave Women*; and Sheridan, *Doctors and Slaves*.
89. Ducoeurjoly, *Manuel des Habitans*.
90. Moitt, "Slave Women and Resistance," 253.
91. Moitt, *Women and Slavery*.

Chapter 4: Enslaved Herbalists

1. Ducoeurjoly, *Manuel des Habitans*, 2: 104.
2. Dutertre, *Histoire Générale*, 2: 409.
3. Shteir, *Cultivating Women*.
4. Gilbert, "Masculine Matrix."
5. Tuana, *Less Noble Sex*.
6. Crespo, "Fragoso, Monardes, and Pre-Chinchonian Knowledge."
7. Ramsey, *Professional and Popular Medicine*.
8. *Affiches Américaines* 22, 1 June 1768, 183. Houghton.
9. Green, *Indigenous Theories*; Mabberley, *Plant-Book*.
10. Iwu, *Handbook*.
11. Dutertre, *Histoire Générale des Antilles*.
12. Charlevoix, *Histoire*; Nau, *Histoire*.
13. Pouppée-Desportes, *Histoire des Maladies*, 3: 59.
14. Antoine de Martinet, *Documents sur les Plantations à Saint Domingue*, 1768–92, AN, T606, Dossier 2.
15. Hall, *Social Control*.
16. Voeks, "African Medicine and Magic."
17. Bourgeois, *Voyages Intéressans*, 503.
18. Debien, *Esclaves aux Antilles*.
19. Hilliard d'Auberteuil, *Considérations*, 1: 219.
20. Dazille, *Observations sur le Tétanos*, 227.
21. For information about the medicinal benefits of cayenne pepper (capsicum), see W. Martin, ed., *Remington's Pharmaceutical Sciences*, 856. I thank Andrew Kovalovich, R.Ph., for calling this information to my attention.
22. Bourgeois, *Voyages Intéressans*, 497, 503. For more information on the medicinal uses of these plants, see Morton, *Atlas*.
23. Pouppée-Desportes, *Histoire des Maladies*, 2: 164.
24. Gardane, *Maladies des Créoles*, 186.
25. Mabberley, *Plant-Book*, 425, 504.

26. Pouppée-Desportes, *Histoire des Maladies*; Goodman, *Tobacco.*
27. Bourgeois, *Voyages Intéressans.*
28. Voeks, "African Medicine and Magic," 75.
29. Dutertre, *Histoire Générale*, 90.
30. Voeks, "African Medicine and Magic."
31. Crespo,"Fragoso, Monardes, and Pre-Chinchonian Knowledge."
32. Morton, *Atlas.*
33. Bourgeois, *Voyages Intéressans.* Geneviève Leti (*Santé et Société*) notes that the effectiveness of the therapies used by slaves in nineteenth-century Martinique were advertised with reference to their having been subjected to experimentation by scientists.
34. Morton, *Atlas.*
35. Bourgeois, *Voyages Intéressans.*
36. Bourgeois, *Voyages Intéressans*, 494–95. Morton states, "It is considered a stimulant and antiscorbutic" (*Atlas*, 364).
37. Gardane, *Maladies des Créoles*, 186.
38. Hippocrates, *Internal Affections*, 52.
39. Bourgeois, *Voyages Intéressans*, 487–89; Arthaud, *Mémoire sur l'Inoculation*, 10.
40. Dazille, *Observations sur le Tétanos*, 312–13.
41. Arthaud, *Observations sur les Lois*, 76.

Chapter 5: Makandal and the Medical Care of Animals

1. Specialists in veterinary medicine have compiled much of the history of veterinary medicine. The historiography of animal medicine has been dedicated to compiling surveys and regional histories. One can easily find studies that concentrate on the rise of veterinary medicine from the prehistoric to the modern periods. See Dunlop and Williams, *Veterinary Medicine*; Karasszon, *Concise History of Veterinary Medicine.* Monographs that focus on particular geographic areas, such as individual states of the United States and specific European nations, are also abundant. Examples of American regional histories are Arnold and Kernkamp, *One Hundred Years*; Dethloff and Dyal, *Special Kind of Doctor.* European national histories include Fisher, "Not Quite a Profession"; Hubscher, "Invention d'une Profession." In addition, scholars have studied the comparative history of human medicine and veterinary medicine. See Mitchell, ed., *History.* Finally, historians have recognized and analyzed the important contributions that slaves in the Roman Empire made to the veterinary sciences. See Dunlop and Williams, *Veterinary Medicine.* The history of veterinary practice by African slaves in the New World, however, has received little attention.
2. Galen, "The Hand."
3. Lovejoy, *Great Chain*; Noske, *Humans*; Peterson, *Being Human*; Sax, *Animals in the Third Reich*; Thomas, *Man and the Natural World.*
4. Hobbes quoted in Worster, *Nature's Economy*, 45.
5. Peterson, *Being Human*, 38–39.
6. Broberg, "Homo Sapiens," 166. Also see Uggla, ed., *Diaeta Naturalis.*
7. Noske, *Humans*; Cooper, *Rousseau and Nature.*
8. Worster, *Nature's Economy.*

9. LaMettrie quoted in Thomas, *Man and the Natural World,* 123; Hume quoted in Thomas, 126. Also see Lovejoy, *Great Chain.*

10. Peterson, *Being Human,* 2.

11. Ibid., 75.

12. Ibid., 2. For an explanation of the "logic of domination," see ibid., 41–44. Also see Thomas, *Man and the Natural World.*

13. My use of the term *myth* takes its inspiration from scholar Charles Bergman, who wrote, "By myth, I do not mean the popular notion of myth as a sort of 'lie.' By myth, I mean the really important that a people or culture elevates to central importance. These stories gain wide currency, last over time. Their value is not that they tell lies, but that they are fictions that define a culture's emotional and psychological truths. These stories become important features of a people's historical and personal experience" (*Orion's Legacy,* 19).

14. Exquemelin, *Buccaneers,* 59.

15. Ibid., 54–55.

16. Bergman, *Orion's Legacy.*

17. Adams, *Sexual Politics.*

18. Moreau de Saint-Méry, *Description Topographique,* 1: 120.

19. Cercle des Philadelphes, *Recherches;* Ducoeurjoly, *Manuel des Habitans;* Laborie, *Coffee Planter.* For secondary source analysis, see Geggus, "Slave and Free Colored Women."

20. Laborie, *Coffee Planter,* 144.

21. Ducoeurjoly, *Manuel des Habitans.*

22. Moreau de Saint-Méry, *Lois et Constitutions.*

23. Dutertre, *Histoire Générale.*

24. McClellan, *Colonialism and Science.*

25. Thomas, *Man and the Natural World.*

26. Quoted in Moitt, "Women, Work, and Resistance," 158. Also see Moitt, *Women and Slavery.*

27. *Gazette de Saint Domingue, Politique, Civile, Economique et Littéraire, et Affiches Américaines,* 12 Nov. 1791, 1037–38. Newberry.

28. Desmangles, *Faces of the Gods,* 31.

29. Ducoeurjoly, *Manuel des Habitans,* 1: 68.

30. Laborie, *Coffee Planter,* 155.

31. Thomas, *Man and the Natural World.*

32. Dayan, *Haiti, History, and the Gods.*

33. Moreau de Saint-Méry, *Description Topographique.* Also see Moitt, "In the Shadow"; Sollors, *Neither Black nor White.*

34. Moreau de Saint-Méry, *Description Topographique,* 1: 119.

35. Cercle des Philadelphes, *Recherches.*

36. Dunlop and Williams, *Veterinary Medicine;* R. O. Gilbert, "Glanders," http://www.vet.uga.edu/vpp/gray_book/Handheld/gla.htm, 7. Accessed 28 June 2002.

37. Moreau de Saint-Méry, *Lois et Constitutions.*

38. Ibid.

39. Ibid.

40. Dunlop and Williams, *Veterinary Medicine.*

41. Karasszon, *Concise History.*

42. Moreau de Saint-Méry, *Description Topographique.*

43. LeCesne, *Correspondance du Gérant*, AN, T561, 16 July 1789, 24 Nov. 1789, 24 Feb. 1790, 8 Apr. 1790.

44. Laborie, *Coffee Planter*. For secondary source information on veterinary handbooks, see Dunlop and Williams, *Veterinary Medicine*.

45. LeCesne, *Correspondance du Gérant*, AN, T561, 28 Jan. 1790.

46. Geggus, "Slave and Free Colored Women"; Laborie, *Coffee Planter*.

47. Laborie, *Coffee Planter*, 166.

48. Karen Davis, "Thinking like a Chicken."

49. Smith and Daniel, *Chicken Book*.

50. Morgan, *Laboring Women*.

51. Bizimana, *Traditional Veterinary Practice*.

52. Ibid.; Smith and Daniel, *Chicken Book*.

53. *Affiches Américaines* 14, 3 Apr. 1781 (suppl.), no page number. Houghton.

54. Laborie, *Coffee Planter*, 98.

55. Cercle des Philadelphes, *Recherches*.

56. Laborie, *Coffee Planter*, 168.

57. Cercle des Philadelphes, *Recherches*; Ducoeurjoly, *Manuel des Habitans*.

58. "Suite du Mémoire sur les Hattes, du Manque de Soins Suffisans au Gouvernement des Bestiaux," *Affiches Américaines*, 6 Apr. 1768, 112. Houghton.

59. LeCesne, *Procuration*, AN, T561, 1 May 1789.

60. *État de l'Habitation de Madame de Chavanne*, AN, T210, Dossier 1, 4 May 1771.

61. Cercle des Philadelphes, *Recherches*; Moitt, "In the Shadow."

62. Laborie, *Coffee Planter*, 179. My emphasis.

63. Monnereau, *Parfait Indigotier*.

64. "Makandal, Histoire Véritable." *Mercure de France*, 15 Sept. 1787, 103. CAOM, BMdSM, 87/MIOM/1.

65. Geggus, *Haitian Revolutionary Studies*.

66. Abdalla, "Islamic Medicine."

67. Imperato, "Traditional African Approaches to Healing."

68. "Makandal, Histoire Véritable"; Moreau de Saint-Méry, *Description Topographique*. Secondary source analyses include Debien, *Esclaves aux Antilles*; Fick, *Making of Haiti*.

69. *Gazette de Saint Domingue, Politique, Civile, Economique et Littéraire, et Affiches Américaines*. 12 Nov. 1791, 1037–38. Newberry.

70. Cauna, "Singularity of the Saint-Domingue Revolution"; Davis, *Serpent and the Rainbow*.

71. Desmangles, *Faces of the Gods*.

72. Moreau de Saint-Méry, *Description Topographique*, 2: 630.

73. "Makandal, Histoire Véritable"; Moreau de Saint-Méry, *Description Topographique*, 2: 630–31.

74. Laurent Dubois, *Avengers*.

75. Ducoeurjoly, *Manuel des Habitans*.

76. Cauna, "Singularity of the Saint-Domingue Revolution."

77. Ducoeurjoly, *Manuel des Habitans*. For secondary source analyses of his name, see Dubois, *Avengers*; Geggus, *Haitian Revolutionary Studies*.

78. Moreau de Saint-Méry, *Lois et Constitutions*; Ducoeurjoly, *Manuel des Habitans*.

79. Moreau de Saint-Méry, *Lois et Constitutions*. For a secondary source analysis of legislation that dealt with poisoning, see Moitt, *Women and Slavery*.

80. Dazille, *Observations sur le Tétanos*, 68.

81. Bertin, *Des Moyens*.

82. Bourgeois, *Voyages Intéressans*; Cercle des Philadelphes, *Recherches*.

83. Girod-Chantrans, *Voyage d'un Suisse*.

84. Hilliard d'Auberteuil, *Considérations*, 139.

85. Moreau de Saint-Méry, *Description Topographique*, 1: 56.

86. Moreau de Saint-Méry, *Lois et Constitutions*, 4: 230.

87. McClellan, *Colonialism and Science*.

88. Hall, *Social Control*.

89. Moreau de Saint-Méry, *Lois et Constitutions*.

90. Cauna, "Singularity of the Saint-Domingue Revolution."

91. Bertin, *Des Moyens*; Pouppée-Desportes, *Histoire des Maladies*; Moreau de Saint-Méry, *Description Topographique*. For secondary source considerations of this issue, see LaGuerre, *Afro-Caribbean Folk Medicine*; McClellan, *Colonialism and Science*.

92. Dubois, *Avengers*.

93. Geggus, *Haitian Revolutionary Studies*.

94. Fick, "French Revolution in Saint Domingue."

95. Cauna, "Singularity of the Saint-Domingue Revolution."

96. Geggus, *Haitian Revolutionary Studies*; Pluchon, *Toussaint Louverture*.

97. Quoted in Pluchon, *Toussaint Louverture*, 58. Also see Pluchon, *Toussaint Louverture de l'Esclavage au Pouvoir*.

98. Dayan, *Haiti, History, and the Gods*; Dubois, *Avengers*; Geggus, *Haitian Revolutionary Studies*; Korngold, *Citizen Toussaint*; Métraux, *Voodoo*; Pluchon, *Toussaint Louverture*; Pluchon, *Toussaint Louverture de l'Esclavage au Pouvoir*; Redpath, *Toussaint L'Ouverture*; Waxman, *Black Napoleon*.

99. Pluchon, *Toussaint Louverture*, 59, 339. Also see Pluchon, *Toussaint Louverture de l'Esclavage au Pouvoir*, 20.

100. Dayan, *Haiti, History, and the Gods*; Dubois, *Avengers*; and Métraux, *Voodoo*.

101. Moitt, *Women and Slavery*.

102. Mullin, *Africa in America*.

Chapter 6: Magnetism in Eighteenth-Century Saint Domingue

1. Modern scholars have seen mesmerism as a lens through which to study, observe, and understand the French Revolution, the transformation of science and medicine in the late eighteenth century, and the development of modern psychiatry. According to Robert Darnton (*Mesmerism*), mesmerism became a rallying point for would-be scholars rejected by the Enlightenment establishment; future French revolutionaries like Jacques-Pierre Brissot and Jean-Louis Carra saw mesmerism as a fight against academic and political despotism. Using gender as an analytical tool, historian Lindsay Wilson (*Women and Medicine*) said that the magnetist debate gave Mesmer's critics opportunities to denounce the dangerous and unnatural control that privileged women had over culture and to proclaim that once women submitted to patriarchal authority, then culture, society, and

the state would be reinvigorated and made healthy. Laurence Brockliss and Colin Jones (*Medical World*) concluded that the mesmerist debate highlighted already existing institutional and epistemological fissures within the medical world of eighteenth-century France. Several authors also have investigated Mesmer's influence on psychiatry, especially his contributions to the practice of hypnotism. Researcher Henri Ellenberger (*Discovery of the Unconscious*) argued that Mesmer advanced the psychological sciences. Similarly, literary scholar Maria M. Tatar ("From Mesmer to Freud") traced the impact that Mesmer and his ideas had on psychoanalysis. Likewise, historian Alan Gauld (*History of Hypnotism*) concluded that Mesmer's striking personality and its impact on several individuals affected the development of psychiatry, psychology, and hypnotism.

2. The dean of Saint Domingue studies, francophone historian Gabriel Debien, traced the history of colonial magnetism in several articles (see "Assemblées Nocturnes," e.g.), and provided transcripts of several key archival sources documenting the incidence of mesmerism. With the exception of historians James McClellan and David Geggus, most anglophone scholars dedicate only a sentence or two to mesmerism in the colony. Examples are Ellenberger, *Discovery of the Unconscious*, 73; Gauld, *A History of Hypnotism*, 39; Geggus, *Haitian Revolutionary Studies*, 79; McClellan, *Colonialism and Science*, 175–80; Wilson, *Women and Medicine*, 122–23.

3. Brockliss and Jones, *Medical World*; Darnton, *Mesmerism*; Gauld, *History of Hypnotism*; Wilson, *Women and Medicine*.

4. Darnton, *Mesmerism*; Gauld, *History of Hypnotism*; Ramsey, *Professional and Popular Medicine*; Wilson, *Women and Medicine*.

5. Gauld, *History of Hypnotism*.

6. Darnton, *Mesmerism*; Wilson, *Women and Medicine*.

7. Ibid.

8. Ibid.

9. McClellan, *Colonialism and Science*.

10. Ibid.

11. Debien, "Profils de Colons," 17. For more information about the research completed by Charles Bonnet, see Magner, *History*.

12. McClellan, *Colonialism and Science*, 177.

13. Ibid.

14. Stein, *French Sugar*, 50.

15. Gauld, *History of Hypnotism*; McClellan, *Colonialism and Science*.

16. Debien, "Profils de Colons," 17.

17. Moreau de Saint-Méry, *Description Topographique*; Debien, "Assemblées Nocturnes."

18. *Extrait des Minutes du Conseil Supérieur du Cap*, AN, 27 AP 12, Dossier 3, 16 May 1786.

19. Cauna, "Singularity of the Saint-Domingue Revolution," 335. Also see Debien, "Assemblées Nocturnes."

20. Moreau de Saint-Méry, *Description Topographique*. Debien provided transcripts of the other two sources in "Document sus les Rites" and "Assemblées Nocturnes."

21. Debien, "Assemblées Nocturnes."

22. Debien, "Document sus les Rites," 73.

23. Moreau de Saint-Méry, *Description Topographique*, 1: 275.

24. Debien, "Assemblées Nocturnes," 277, 279, 280.
25. Ibid., 279.
26. Moreau de Saint-Méry, *Lois et Constitutions.*
27. Debien, "Assemblées Nocturnes," 279.
28. Ibid.
29. Moreau de Saint-Méry, *Description Topographique,* 1: 275.
30. Debien, "Assemblées Nocturnes," 281.
31. Debien, "Document sus les Rites."
32. Debien, "Assemblées Nocturnes," 279.
33. Debien, "Document sus les Rites."
34. Moreau de Saint-Méry, *Description Topographique.*
35. Debien, "Assemblées Nocturnes."
36. Moreau de Saint-Méry, *Description Topographique,* 1: 276.
37. Debien, "Assemblées Nocturnes," 282–83.
38. Ibid.
39. Ibid., 277.
40. Métraux, *Voodoo,* 11–12.
41. Brown, *Mama Lola;* Desmangles, *Faces of the Gods.*
42. Debien, "Assemblées Nocturnes."
43. Moreau de Saint-Méry, *Description Topographique.* For secondary source analyses, see Debien, "Document sus les Rites"; Geggus, *Haitian Revolutionary Studies;* Métraux, *Voodoo.*
44. Deren, *Divine Horsemen.*
45. Desmangles, *Faces of the Gods,* 121.
46. Ellenberger, *Discovery of the Unconscious.*

Chapter 7: The Transformative Power of the Kaperlata

1. The story of the *kaperlata*s has received little attention from historians of eighteenth-century Saint Domingue, especially anglophone scholars. The most recent reference in any language to the *kaperlata*s came from James E. McClellan (*Colonialism and Science*), who noted their illegality and the fear they inspired among white colonists. The most thorough study of these enslaved healers was the work of Pierre Pluchon (*Vaudou Sorciers*), who considered them within the context of European fears about sorcery and French colonial efforts to stamp out the practice of what they perceived as magical medicine.
2. *Kingué (sur les Méfaits de),* AN, 27 AP 12, Dossier 2, 1785.
3. Peek, *African Divination Systems.*
4. Moreau de Saint-Méry, *Description Topographique,* 1: 56.
5. *Kingué (sur les Méfaits de),* AN, 27 AP 12, Dossier 2, 1785.
6. Durkheim and Mauss quoted in Peek, *African Divination Systems,* 6.
7. Moreau de Saint-Méry, *Description Topographique,* 1: 56. For a secondary source analysis, see Hall, *Social Control.*
8. Raboteau, *Slave Religion.*
9. *Kingué (sur les Méfaits de),* AN, 27 AP 12, Dossier 2, 1785. For a discussion of Kingué, see Pluchon, *Vaudou Sorciers.*
10. Ramsey, *Professional and Popular Medicine.*
11. Ibid.

12. Bush, *Slave Women.*
13. Cohen, *French Encounter.*
14. Ibid., 17. For English attitudes toward Africans, see Jordan, *White over Black.*
15. Moreau de Saint-Méry, *Description Topographique,* 1: 56.
16. *Kingué (sur les Méfaits de),* AN, 27 AP 12, Dossier 2, 1785.
17. Moreau de Saint-Méry, *Description Topographique,* 1: 90.
18. Arthaud, *Observations sur les Lois.*
19. Ibid, 77.
20. Ibid.
21. Plato, *Republic.*
22. Eliot, ed., *Folklore and Fable.* For a discussion of Greek and Roman contributions to the notion of the body politic, see Hale, *Body Politic.*
23. Kantorowicz, *King's Two Bodies;* Melzer and Norberg, *From the Royal to the Republican Body.*
24. Hobbes, *Leviathan.*
25. Jean-Jacques Rousseau, *Social Contract.* For a discussion of social contract theory and the transformation of the body politic, see Hale, *Body Politic;* Landes, *Visualizing the Nation.*
26. Hobbes's description is on 247–57 of *Leviathan* and Rousseau's is on 76–80 of *Social Contract.*
27. Brockliss and Jones, *Medical World.*
28. Ibid.
29. Baecque, *Body Politic.*
30. *Extrait des Minutes du Conseil Supérieur du Cap,* AN, 27 AP 12, Dossier 3, 16 May 1786.
31. Descourtilz, *Histoire des Désastres,* 103.
32. Bush, *Slave Women;* Debien, *Esclaves aux Antilles;* Fick, *Making of Haiti;* Hall, *Social Control.*
33. Moreau de Saint-Méry, *Description Topographique.*
34. Moitt, *Women and Slavery;* Morrisey, *Slave Women.*
35. Edwards, *Historical Survey.*
36. Ibid., xx, 80, 82; also see Descourtilz, *Histoire des Désastres.*
37. Davis, *Passage of Darkness.*
38. Moreau de Saint-Méry, *Description Topographique,* 1: 64.

Conclusion

1. Lans, *Creole Remedies;* Tarbes, "Cross-Cultural Ethnomedical Research"; Elisabetsky and de Moraes, "Ethnopharmacology."

BIBLIOGRAPHY

Archival Sources

Note: Translations of archival materials in the text and notes are my own.

Andruss Library, Bloomsburg University, Bloomsburg, Pa. Cited as Bloomsburg.
Archives Nationales, Paris. Cited as AN.
Archives Nationales: Section d'Outre-Mer, Aix-en-Provence. Cited as CAOM.
Bibliothèque Moreau de Saint-Méry, Archives Nationales: Section d'Outre-Mer, Aix-en-Provence. Cited as CAOM, BMdSM.
College of Physicians of Philadelphia.
Hagley Museum and Library, Archives and Manuscripts Department, Wilmington, Delaware. Cited as Hagley.
Haverford College Library, Quaker Collection, Haverford, Pa. Cited as Haverford.
Houghton Library, Harvard University, Cambridge, Mass. Cited as Houghton.
Newberry Library, Chicago. Cited as Newberry.
Pattee Library, Pennsylvania State University, University Park, Pa. Cited as Pattee.
Van Pelt-Dietrich Library Center, Department of Special Collections, University of Pennsylvania, Philadelphia, Pa. Cited as Van Pelt.
Wellcome Library for the History and Understanding of Medicine, London. Cited as Wellcome.

Published Material

Abdalla, Ismail Hussein. "Islamic Medicine and Its Influence on Traditional Hausa Practitioners in Northern Nigeria." Ph.D. diss., University of Wisconsin–Madison, 1981.
Ackerknecht, Erwin H. *A Short History of Medicine.* Rev. ed. Baltimore: Johns Hopkins University Press, 1982.
Adams, Carol J. *The Sexual Politics of Meat: A Feminist-Vegetarian Critical Theory.* New York: Continuum, 1990.
Altema, Reynald, and Leslie Bright. "Letter to the Editor: Only Homosexual Haitians, Not All Haitians." *Annals of Internal Medicine* 99 (Dec. 1983): 877–78.
Arnold, David, ed. *Imperial Medicine and Indigenous Societies.* Manchester, U.K.: Manchester University Press, 1988.
———. *Warm Climates and Western Medicine.* Amsterdam, Neth.: Rodopi, 1996.
Arnold, John P., and H. C. H. Kernkamp. *One Hundred Years of Progress: The History of Veterinary Medicine in Minnesota.* St. Paul, Minn.: Minnesota Veterinary Historical Museum, 1994.

Arthaud, Charles. Discours prononcé à l'ouverture de la première séance publique du Cercle des Philadelphes, tenue au Cap-François le 11 Mai 1785. Cap-François, 11 Mai 1785. CAOM, 87/M10M/44, BMdSM. Text-fiche.

———. *Mémoire sur l'Inoculation de la Petite Vérole.* Cap-François, 1774. CAOM, 87/MIOM/63. Text-fiche.

———. *Observations sur les Lois, concernant la Médecine et la Chirurgie dans la Colonie de St. Domingue, avec des Vues de Règlement, Adressées au Comité du Salubrité de l'Assemblée Nationale et à l'Assemblée Coloniale,* Cap-François, 1791, CAOM, 87/MIOM/41. Text-fiche.

Arthaud, Charles, and J. Cosme D'Angerville, *Procès Verbal de Visite des Prisons Royales du Cap,* AN, 27 AP 11, Dossier 3, 22 Dec. 1786.

Baecque, Antoine de. *The Body Politic: Corporeal Metaphor in Revolutionary France, 1770–1800.* Translated by Charlotte Mandell. Stanford, Calif.: Stanford University Press, 1997.

Bankole, Katherine. *Slavery and Medicine: Enslavement and Medical Practices in Antebellum Louisiana.* New York: Garland, 1998.

Barry, Michelle, John Mellors, and Frank Bia. "Haiti and the AIDS Connection." *Journal of Chronic Diseases* 37 (1984): 593–95.

Beckles, Hilary M. *Natural Rebels: A Social History of Enslaved Black Women in Barbados.* New Brunswick, N.J.: Rutgers University Press, 1989.

Bergman, Charles. *Orion's Legacy: A Cultural History of Man as Hunter.* New York: Dutton, 1996.

Bertin, N. *Des Moyens de Conserver la Santé des Blancs et des Nègres aux Antilles ou Climats Chauds.* Paris, 1786. Haverford.

Bizimana, Nsekuye. *Traditional Veterinary Practice in Africa.* Eschborn, Ger.: Deutsche Gesellschaft für Technische Zusammenarbeit, 1994.

Boncy, Madeleine, A. Claude LaRoche, Bernard Liautaud, Jean-Robert Mathurin, Jean William Pape, Molière Pamphile, Vergniaud Péan, Marie-Myrtha St-Amand, Franck Thomas, Emmanuel Arnoux, Robert Elie, Jean-Michel Guérin, Rodolphe Malebranche, and Gérard Pierre. "Letter to the Editor: Acquired Immunodeficiency in Haitians." *New England Journal of Medicine* 308 (9 June 1983): 1419–20.

Bordes, Ary. *Évolution des Sciences, de la Santé et de l'Hygiène Publique en Haïti.* Vol. 1: *Fin de la Période Coloniale-1915.* Port-au-Prince, Haïti: Centre d'Hygiène Familiale, 1979.

Bourgeois, Nicolas Louis. *Voyages Intéressans dans Différentes Colonies Françaises, Espagnoles, Anglaises, &c.* London, 1788. College of Physicians of Philadelphia.

Broberg, Gunnar. "*Homo Sapiens.* Linnaeus's Classification of Man." In *Linnaeus: The Man and His Work,* ed. Tore Frangsmyr, 156–94. Berkeley: University of California Press, 1983.

Brockliss, Laurence, and Colin Jones. *The Medical World of Early Modern France.* Oxford, U.K.: Clarendon Press, 1997.

Brown, Jonathan. *The History and Present Condition of St. Domingo.* Philadelphia: William Marshall, 1837.

Brown, Karen McCarthy. *Mama Lola: A Vodou Priestess in Brooklyn.* Berkeley: University of California Press, 1991.

Bush, Barbara. *Slave Women in Caribbean Society, 1650–1838.* Bloomington: Indiana University Press, 1990.

Butler, Charles S. "Some Contributions of United States Naval Medical Officers to Science." *American Journal of Tropical Medicine* 21 (1941): 23. College of Physicians of Philadelphia.

Cauna, Jacques. *Au Temps des Isles à Sucre: Histoire d'une Plantation de Saint-Domingue au XVIIIᵉSiècle.* Paris: Éditions Karthala, 1987.

———. "The Singularity of the Saint-Domingue Revolution: Marronage, Voodoo, and the Color Question." *Plantation Society in the Americas* 3 (1996): 321–45.

Cercle des Philadelphes. *Recherches, Mémoires et Observations sur les Maladies Épizootiques de Saint Domingue.* Cap-François, 1788. College of Physicians of Philadelphia.

Chandler, Asa, and Clark Read. *Introduction to Parasitology.* New York: Wiley & Sons, 1961.

Charlevoix, Pierre-François-Xavier. *Histoire de l'Isle Espagnole ou de S. Domingue. . . .* Paris, 1730. Hagley.

Chevalier, Jean-Damien. *Lettres à M. de Jean, Docteur-Régent de la Faculté de Médecine, en l'Université de Paris. . . .* Paris, 1752. College of Physicians of Philadelphia.

Cineas, Fritz N. "Letter to the Editor: Haitian Ambassador Deplores AIDS Connections." *New England Journal of Medicine* 309 (15 Sept. 1983): 668–69.

Cohen, William B. *The French Encounter with Africans: White Response to Blacks, 1530–1880.* Bloomington: Indiana University Press, 1980.

College of Physicians of Philadelphia. *Facts and Observations Relative to the Nature and Origin of the Pestilential Fever, Which Prevailed in this City, in 1793, 1794, 1797, and 1798.* Philadelphia, 1798. Pattee. Text-fiche.

Cooper, Laurence D. *Rousseau and Nature: The Problem of the Good Life.* University Park, Pa.: Pennsylvania State University Press, 1999.

Crespo, Fernando I. Ortíz. "Fragoso, Monardes, and Pre-Chinchonian Knowledge of Cinchona." *Archives of Natural History* 22 (1995): 169–81.

Cunningham, Andrew, and Roger French, eds. *The Medical Enlightenment of the Eighteenth Century.* Cambridge, U.K.: Cambridge University Press, 1990.

Currie, William. *A Description of the Malignant Infectious Fever Prevailing at Present in Philadelphia.* Philadelphia, 1793. Pattee. Text-fiche.

———. *An Impartial Review of That Part of Dr. Rush's Late Publication.* Philadelphia, 1794. Pattee. Text-fiche.

Darnton, Robert. *Mesmerism and the End of the Enlightenment in France.* Cambridge, Mass.: Harvard University Press, 1968.

Davis, Karen. "Thinking like a Chicken: Farm Animals and the Feminine Connection." In *Animals and Women: Feminist Theoretical Explorations,* ed. Carol J. Adams and Josephine Donovan, 192–212. Durham, N.C.: Duke University Press, 1995.

Davis, Wade. *Passage of Darkness: The Ethnobiology of the Haitian Zombie.* Chapel Hill: University of North Carolina Press, 1988.

———. *The Serpent and the Rainbow.* New York: Warner Books, 1985.

Dayan, Joan. *Haiti, History, and the Gods.* Berkeley: University of California Press, 1995.

Dazille, Jean-Barthélemy. *Observations sur la Santé des Femmes Enceintes entre les Tropiques.* Paris, 1788. College of Physicians of Philadelphia.

———. *Observations sur les Maladies des Nègres, Leurs Causes, Leurs Traitemens et les Moyens de Les Prévenir.* Paris, 1776. College of Physicians of Philadelphia.

———. *Observations sur le Tétanos*. Paris, 1788. College of Physicians of Philadelphia.

Debien, Gabriel. "Assemblées Nocturnes d'Esclaves à Saint Domingue." *Annales Historiques de la Révolution Française* 44 (1972): 273–84.

———. *Les Esclaves aux Antilles Françaises (XVII–XVIIIᵉSiècles)*. Basse-Terre, Guadaloupe: Société d'Histoire de la Guadeloupe, 1974.

———. *Plantations et Esclaves à Saint Domingue*. Dakar, Senegal: Université de Dakar, 1962.

———. "Profils de Colons: Jean Trembley." *Revue de la Porte Océane* 11 (1955): 14–19.

———. "Un Document sus les Rites Secrets des Nègres à Saint-Domingue." *Revue de l'Histoire des Colonies Françaises* 22 (1929): 72–74.

Délorme. "Reflexions sur la Topographie Médicale du Cap, par le Citoyen Délorme, Chirurgien en Chef de l'Hôpital Durand." *Journal des Officiers de Santé de Saint Domingue* 1 (1803): 2. Wellcome.

Deren, Maya. *Divine Horsemen: Voodoo Gods of Haiti*. New York: Chelsea House, 1970.

Desmangles, Leslie G. *The Faces of the Gods: Vodou & Roman Catholicism in Haiti*. Chapel Hill: University of North Carolina Press, 1992.

Descourtilz, Michel-Étienne. *Histoire des Désastres de Saint-Domingue. . . .* Paris, 1795. Van Pelt.

Dethloff, Henry C., and Donald H. Dyal. *A Special Kind of Doctor: A History of Veterinary Medicine in Texas*. College Station: Texas A&M University Press, 1991.

Dubois, Laurent. *Avengers of the New World: The Story of the Haitian Revolution*. Cambridge, Mass.: Belknap Press, 2004.

Ducoeurjoly, S. J. *Manuel des Habitans de Saint-Domingue*. Paris, 1802. Newberry.

Dunlop, Robert H., and David J. Williams. *Veterinary Medicine: An Illustrated History*. St. Louis, Mo.: Mosby-Year Book, 1996.

Dutertre, Jean-Baptiste. *Histoire Générale des Antilles*. 4 vols. Paris, 1667. Newberry.

Edwards, Bryan. *An Historical Survey of the French Colony in the Island of St. Domingo*. London, 1797. Pattee.

Eliot, Charles W., ed. *Folklore and Fable: Aesop, Grimm, and Andersen*. New York: Collier, 1909.

Elisabetsky, Elaine, and João A. R. de Moraes. "Ethnopharmacology: A Technological Development Strategy." In *Ethnobiology: Implications and Applications*. Proceedings of the First International Congress of Ethnobiology, ed. Darrell A. Posey and William Leslie Overal, 111–23. Belém, Brazil: Museu Paraense Emílio Goeldi, 1988.

Ellenberger, Henri F. *The Discovery of the Unconscious: The History and Evolution of Dynamic Psychiatry*. New York: Basic Books, 1970.

Exquemelin, Alexander O. *The Buccaneers of America*. Translated by Alexis Brown. Baltimore: Penguin Books, 1969.

Farmer, Paul. *AIDS and Accusation: Haiti and the Geography of Blame*. Berkeley: University of California Press, 1992.

Fenner, Frank, Donald A. Henderson, Isao Arita, Zdenek Ježek, and Ivan Danilovich Ladnyi. *Smallpox and Its Eradication*. Geneva, Switz.: World Health Organization, 1988.

Fick, Carolyn. "The French Revolution in Saint Domingue: A Triumph or Failure?" In *A Turbulent Time: The French Revolution and the Greater Caribbean,* ed. David Barry Gaspar and David Patrick Geggus, 51–75. Bloomington: Indiana University Press, 1997.

———. *The Making of Haiti: The Saint Domingue Revolution from Below.* Knoxville: University of Tennessee Press, 1990.

Fisher, J. R. "Not Quite a Profession: The Aspirations of Veterinary Surgeons in England in the Mid-Nineteenth Century." *Historical Research* 66 (1993): 284–302.

Galen. "The Hand." In *Medicine and Western Civilization,* ed. David J. Rothman, Steven Marcus, and Stephanie A. Kiceluk, 17–22. New Brunswick, N.J.: Rutgers University Press, 1995.

Gardane, Joseph Jacques de. *Des Maladies des Créoles en Europe.* Paris, 1786. College of Physicians of Philadelphia.

Gauld, Alan. *A History of Hypnotism.* Cambridge, U.K.: Cambridge University Press, 1992.

Gautier, Arlette. *Les Soeurs de Solitude: La Condition Féminine dans l'Esclavage aux Antilles du XVIIᵉ au XIXᵉ Siècle.* Paris: Éditions Caribéenes, 1985.

Geggus, David Patrick. *Haitian Revolutionary Studies.* Bloomington: Indiana University Press, 2002.

———. "Slave and Free Colored Women in Saint Domingue." In *More Than Chattel: Black Women and Slavery in the Americas,* ed. David Barry Gaspar and Darlene Clark Hine, 259–78. Bloomington: Indiana University Press, 1996.

Gelfand, Toby. "A 'Monarchical Profession' in the Old Regime: Surgeons, Ordinary Practitioners, and Medical Professionalization in Eighteenth-Century France." In *Professions and the French State, 1700–1900,* ed. Gerald L. Geison, 149–80. Philadelphia: University of Pennsylvania Press, 1984.

Gilbert, R. O. "Glanders." http://www.vet.uga.edu/vpp/gray_book/Handheld/gla.htm, 7. Accessed 28 June 2002.

Gilbert, Ruth. "The Masculine Matrix: Male Births and the Scientific Imagination in Early Modern England." In *The Arts of 17th-Century Science: Representations of the Natural World in European and North American Culture,* ed. Claire Jowitt and Diane Watt, 160–75. Hants, U.K.: Ashgate, 2002.

Girod-Chantrans, Justin. *Voyage d'un Suisse dans Différentes Colonies d'Amérique pendant la Dernière Guerre. . . .* Neuchâtel, 1785. Hagley.

Goodman, Jordan. *Tobacco in History: The Cultures of Dependence.* New York: Routledge, 1993.

Greco, Ralph S. "Letter to the Editor: Haiti and the Stigma of AIDS." *Lancet* 2 (27 Aug. 1983): 515–16.

Green, Edward C. *Indigenous Theories of Contagious Disease.* Walnut Creek, Calif.: AltaMira Press, 1999.

Hale, David George. *The Body Politic: A Political Metaphor in Renaissance English Literature.* Paris: Mouton, 1971.

Hall, Gwendolyn Mildo. *Social Control in Slave Plantation Societies: A Comparison of St. Domingue and Cuba.* Baton Rouge: Louisiana State University Press, 1971.

Herbert, Eugenia W. "Smallpox Inoculation in Africa." *Journal of African History* 16, 4 (1975): 547–48.

Hilliard d'Auberteuil, Michel-René. *Considérations sur l'État Présent de la Colonie Française de Saint Domingue, Ouvrage Politique et Législatif.* Paris, 1776. Hagley.

Hippocrates. *Internal Affections.* Translated by Paul Potter. Cambridge, Mass.: Harvard University Press, 1988.

Hobbes, Thomas. *Leviathan, or the Matter, Forme, & Power of a Commonwealth Ecclesiasticall and Civill.* London, 1651; repr., Oxford, U.K.: Clarendon Press, 1967.

Hopkins, Donald. *Princes and Peasants: Smallpox in History.* Chicago: University of Chicago Press, 1983.

Hubscher, Ronald. "L'Invention d'une Profession: Les Vétérinaires au XIXᵉ Siècle." *Revue d'Histoire Moderne et Contemporaine* 43 (1996): 686–708.

Imperato, Pascal James. "Traditional African Approaches to Healing." *Caduceus* 9 (1993): 17–36.

Isert, Paul Erdman, *Voyages en Guinée et dans les Iles Caraïbes en Amérique. Translaté de l'allemand,* Paris, 1793, CAOM, 87/MIOM/15, BMdSM. Textfiche.

Iwu, Maurice M. *Handbook of African Medicinal Plants.* Boca Raton, Fla.: CRC Press, 1993.

James, C. L. R. *The Black Jacobins: Toussaint L'Ouverture and the San Domingo Revolution.* 2d ed., rev. New York: Vintage Books, 1963.

James, Preston E., and Geoffrey J. Martin. *All Possible Worlds: A History of Geographical Ideas.* 2d ed. New York: Wiley & Sons, 1972.

Jordan, Winthrop D. *White over Black: American Attitudes toward the Negro, 1550–1812.* Chapel Hill: University of North Carolina Press, 1979.

Kantorowicz, Ernst. *The King's Two Bodies: A Study in Mediaeval Political Theology.* Princeton, N.J.: Princeton University Press, 1957.

Karasszon, Dénes. *A Concise History of Veterinary Medicine.* Translated by Iringo K. Kecskés. Budapest, Hungary: Akadémiai Kiadó, 1988.

Kiple, Kenneth. *The African Exchange: Toward a Biological History of Black People.* Durham, N.C.: Duke University Press, 1987.

———. *The Caribbean Slave: A Biological History.* Cambridge, U.K.: Cambridge University Press, 1984.

Kiple, Kenneth F., ed. *The Cambridge World History.* Cambridge, U.K.: Cambridge University Press, 1993.

Kiple, Kenneth F., and Virginia Himmelsteib King. *Another Dimension to the Black Diaspora: Diet, Disease, and Racism.* Cambridge, U.K.: Cambridge University Press, 1981.

Korngold, Ralph. *Citizen Toussaint.* New York: Hill and Wang, 1965.

Labat, Jean-Baptiste. *Nouveau Voyage aux Isles de l'Amérique.* 3 vols. The Hague, 1724. Pattee. Text-fiche.

Laborie, J. *The Coffee Planter of Saint Domingue.* London, 1798. Newberry.

Lafosse, J. F. *Avis aux Habitans des Colonies, Particulièrement à Ceux de l'Isle S. Domingue. . . .* Paris, 1787. CAOM, 87/MIOM/4.

LaGuerre, Michel. *Afro-Caribbean Folk Medicine.* South Hadley, Mass.: Bergen and Garvey, 1987.

Landes, Joan. *Visualizing the Nation: Gender, Representation, and Revolution in Eighteenth-Century France.* Ithaca, N.Y.: Cornell University Press, 2001.

Lans, Cheryl. "Creole Remedies: Case Studies of Ethnoveterinary Medicine in Trinidad and Tobago." Unpublished Ph.D. thesis, Wageningen Universiteit, Holland, 2001. Purdue University Library.

Lenman, Bruce P. "Colonial Wars and Imperial Instability, 1688–1793," In *The*

Eighteenth Century, vol. 2, ed. P. J. Marshall, 151–67. Oxford, U.K.: Oxford University Press, 1998.

Léon, Rulx. "Une Esquisse de l'Histoire de la Médecine en Haïti." *Conjonction* 47 (1953): 5–17.

Leonidas, Jean-Robert, and Nicole Hyppolite. "Haiti and the Acquired Immunodeficiency Syndrome." *Annals of Internal Medicine* 98 (June 1983): 1020–21.

Leti, Geneviève. *Santé et Société Esclavagiste à la Martinique*. Paris: Éditions L'Harmattan, 1998.

Lewis, Gordon K. *Main Currents in Caribbean Thought: The Historical Evolutions of Caribbean Society in Its Ideological Aspects, 1492–1900*. Baltimore: Johns Hopkins University Press, 1983.

Livingstone, David N. *The Geographical Tradition: Episodes in the History of a Contested Enterprise*. Cambridge, Mass.: Blackwell, 1993.

Lovejoy, Arthur O. *The Great Chain of Being: A Study of the History of an Idea*. New York: Harper Torchbooks, 1960.

Mabberley, D. J. *The Plant-Book: A Portable Dictionary of the Higher Plants*. Cambridge, U.K.: Cambridge University Press, 1987.

Magner, Lois. *A History of the Life Sciences*. 2d ed. New York: Marcel Dekker, 1994.

Martin, Eric W., ed. *Remington's Pharmaceutical Sciences*. 13th ed. Easton, Pa.: Mack, 1965.

Marx, Jean. "Acquired Immune Deficiency Syndrome Abroad." *Science* 222 (2 Dec. 1983): 998–99.

McClellan, James E. III. *Colonialism and Science: Saint Domingue in the Old Regime*. Baltimore: Johns Hopkins University Press, 1992.

McClellan, James E. III, and François Regourd. "The Colonial Machine: French Science and Colonization in the Ancien Régime." *Osiris* 15 (2000): 31–50.

Melzer, Sara E., and Kathryn Norberg. *From the Royal to the Republican Body: Incorporating the Political in Seventeenth- and Eighteenth-Century France*. Berkeley: University of California Press, 1998.

Métraux, Alfred. *Voodoo in Haiti*. Translated by Hugo Chartiers. New York: Schocken Books, 1972.

Mintz, Sidney W. "Slave Life in Caribbean Sugar Plantations: Some Unanswered Questions." In *Slave Cultures and the Cultures of Slavery*, ed. Stephan Palmie, 12–22. Knoxville: University of Tennessee Press, 1995.

Mitchell, A. R., ed. *History of the Healing Professions: Parallels between Veterinary and Medical History*. Wallingford, U.K.: CAB International, 1993.

Moitt, Bernard. "In the Shadow of the Plantation: Women of Color and the *Libres de Fait* of Martinique and Guadeloupe, 1658–1848." In *Beyond Bondage: Free Women of Color in the Americas*, ed. Darlene Clark Hine and David Barry Gaspar, 37–59. Urbana: University of Illinois Press, 2004.

———. "Slave Women and Resistance in the French Caribbean." In *More Than Chattel: Black Women and Slavery in the Americas*, ed. David Barry Gaspar and Darlene Clark Hine, 239–58. Bloomington: Indiana University Press, 1996.

———. *Women and Slavery in the French Antilles, 1635–1845*. Bloomington: Indiana University Press, 2001.

———. "Women, Work, and Resistance in the French Caribbean during Slavery, 1700–1848." In *Engendering History: Caribbean Women in Historical Perspective*, ed. Verene Shepherd, Bridget Brereton, and Barbara Bailey, 155–75. New York: St. Martin's Press, 1995.

Monnereau, Élie. *Le Parfait Indigotier.* Marseille, 1765. Hagley.

Montesquieu, Charles-Louis de Secondat, baron de. *The Spirit of the Laws.* Translated and edited by Anne M. Cohler, Basia Carolyn Miller, and Harold Samuel Stone. Cambridge, U.K.: Cambridge University Press, 1989. [Originally published 1758.]

Moreau de Saint-Méry, Médéric-Louis-Élie. *Description Topographique, Physique, Civile, Politique et Historique de la Partie Française de l'Isle Saint-Domingue.* Philadelphia, 1797; repr., Paris: Société de l'Histoire des Colonies Françaises, 1958. Pattee.

———. *Lois et Constitutions.* 6 vols. Paris, 1784–1790. Newberry.

Morgan, Jennifer. *Laboring Women: Reproduction and Gender in New World Slavery.* Philadelphia: University of Pennsylvania Press, 2004.

Morgan, Philip D. *Slave Counterpoint: Black Culture in the Eighteenth-Century Chesapeake and Lowcountry.* Omohundro Institute of Early American History and Culture. Chapel Hill: University of North Carolina Press, 1998.

Morrissey, Marietta. *Slave Women in the New World: Gender Stratification in the Caribbean.* Lawrence: University of Kansas Press, 1989.

Morton, Julia F. *Atlas of the Medicinal Plants of Middle America: Bahamas to Yucatan.* Springfield, Ill.: Charles C. Thomas, 1981.

Moses, Peter, and John Moses. "Letter to the Editor: Haiti and the Acquired Immunodeficiency Syndrome." *Annals of Internal Medicine* 99 (Oct. 1983): 565.

Mullin, Michael. *Africa in America: Slave Acculturation and Resistance in the American South and the British Caribbean, 1736–1831.* Urbana: University of Illinois Press, 1992.

Nau, Émile. *Histoire des Caciques d'Haiti.* Port-au-Prince, Haiti: T. Bouchereau, 1855. Text-fiche. Bloomsburg.

Noske, Barbara. *Humans and Other Animals: Beyond the Boundaries of Anthropology.* Winchester, Mass.: Pluto Press, 1989.

Nussbaum, Felicity A. *Torrid Zones: Maternity, Sexuality, and Empire in Eighteenth-Century English Narratives.* Baltimore: Johns Hopkins University Press, 1995.

Peek, Philip M., ed. *African Divination Systems: Ways of Knowing.* Bloomington: Indiana University Press, 1990.

Peterson, Anna L. *Being Human: Ethics, Environment, and Our Place in the World.* Berkeley: University of California Press, 2001.

Pluchon, Pierre. *Toussaint Louverture: Un Révolutionnaire Noir d'Ancien Régime.* Paris: Fayard, 1989.

———. *Toussaint Louverture de l'Esclavage au Pouvoir.* Paris: l'École, 1979.

———. *Vaudou Sorciers Empoisonneurs de Saint-Domingue à Haïti.* Paris: Karthala, 1987.

Pluchon, Pierre, ed. *Histoire des Médecins et Pharmaciens de Marine et des Colonies.* Toulouse, Fr.: Privat, 1985.

Poisonnier-Desperrières, Antoine. *Traité des Fièvres de l'Ile de Saint-Domingue.* Paris, 1766. College of Physicians of Philadelphia.

———. *Traité sur les Maladies des Gens de Mer.* Paris, 1767. College of Physicians of Philadelphia.

Porter, Roy, ed. *The Cambridge Illustrated History of Medicine.* Cambridge: Cambridge University Press, 1996.

Pouppée-Desportes, Jean-Baptiste-René. *Histoire des Maladies de S. Domingue* 3 vols. Paris, 1770. College of Physicians of Philadelphia.

Raboteau, Albert J. *Slave Religion: The "Invisible Institution" in the Antebellum South.* New York: Oxford University Press, 1978.

Ramsey, Matthew. *Professional and Popular Medicine in France, 1770–1830: The Social World of Medical Practice.* Cambridge, U.K.: Cambridge University Press, 1988.

Raynal, Guillaume. *Essai sur l'administration de St. Domingue.* N.P., 1785. Newberry

Redpath, James. *Toussaint L'Ouverture: A Biography and Autobiography.* Boston: James Redpath, 1863; repr., Salem, N.H.: Ayer, 1991.

Rousseau, Jean-Jacques. *The Social Contract.* Translated by Charles Frankel. New York: Hafner, 1947.

Savitt, Todd L. *Medicine and Slavery: The Diseases and Health Care of Blacks in Antebellum Virginia.* Urbana: University of Illinois Press, 1978.

Sax, Boria. *Animals in the Third Reich: Pets, Scapegoats, and the Holocaust.* New York: Continuum Books, 2000.

Schiebinger, Londa. *The Mind Has No Sex? Women in the Origins of Modern Science.* Cambridge, Mass.: Harvard University Press, 1989.

Scott, James C. *Domination and the Arts of Resistance: Hidden Transcripts.* New Haven, Conn.: Yale University Press, 1990.

Sheridan, Richard. *Doctors and Slaves: A Medical and Demographic History of Slavery in the British West Indies, 1680–1834.* Cambridge, U.K.: Cambridge University Press, 1985.

Shteir, Ann B. *Cultivating Women, Cultivating Science.* Baltimore: Johns Hopkins University Press, 1996.

Smith, Page, and Charles Daniel. *The Chicken Book.* San Francisco: North Point Press, 1982.

Sollors, Werner. *Neither Black nor White yet Both: Thematic Explorations of Interracial Literature.* New York: Oxford University Press, 1997.

Stannard, David E. *American Holocaust: Columbus and the Conquest of the New World.* New York: Oxford University Press, 1992.

Stein, Robert Louis. *The French Sugar Business in the Eighteenth Century.* Baton Rouge: Louisiana State University Press, 1988.

Stewart, Larry. "The Edge of Utility: Slaves and Smallpox in the Early Eighteenth Century." *Medical History* 29, 1 (1985): 54–70.

Tarbes, María G. González. "On Cross-Cultural Ethnomedical Research." *Current Anthropology* 30, 1 (1989): 75–76.

Tatar, Maria M. "From Mesmer to Freud: Animal Magnetism, Hypnosis, and Suggestion." In *Spellbound: Studies on Mesmerism and Literature,* ed. Maria M. Tatar, 3–44. Princeton, N.J.: Princeton University Press, 1978.

Thomas, Keith. *Man and the Natural World: A History of the Modern Sensibility.* New York: Pantheon Books, 1983.

Tuana, Nancy. *The Less Noble Sex: Scientific, Religious, and Philosophical Conceptions of Women's Nature.* Bloomington: Indiana University Press, 1993.

Uggla, A. H., ed. *Diaeta Naturalis.* Stockholm, n.p.: 1957. [Originally published in 1733.]

"Update on Acquired Immune Deficiency Syndrome (AIDS)—United States." *MMWR* 31 (1982): 507–14.

Vaughan, Megan. "Slavery, Smallpox, and Revolution: 1792 in Ile-de-France." *Social History of Medicine* 13 (2000): 411–28.

Voeks, Robert. "African Medicine and Magic." *Geographical Review* 83, 1 (1993): 66–79.

Waxman, Percy. *The Black Napoleon: The Story of Toussaint Louverture.* New York: Harcourt, Brace, 1931.

Wilson, Lindsay. *Women and Medicine in the French Enlightenment: The Debate over Maladies des Femmes.* Baltimore: Johns Hopkins University Press, 1993.

Winslow, Ola Elizabeth. *A Destroying Angel: The Conquest of Smallpox in Colonial Boston.* Boston: Houghton Mifflin, 1974.

Worster, Donald. *Nature's Economy: The Roots of Ecology.* San Francisco: Sierra Club Books, 1977.

INDEX

Page numbers in italics refer to pages with illustrations.

KAROL K. WEAVER is an assistant professor of
history and the Winifred and Gustave Weber Fellow
in the Humanities at Susquehanna University. She
has published articles in *Bulletin of the History of
Medicine, French Colonial History, Nursing History
Review,* and *Pennsylvania History.* She was a Camargo
Fellow in fall 1998.

The University of Illinois Press
is a founding member of the
Association of American University Presses.

University of Illinois Press
1325 South Oak Street
Champaign, IL 61820-6903
www.press.uillinois.edu